Suck It Breast Cancer Coloring Book

© 2018 Pink Ribbon Colorists

All Rights Reserved.

This book or parts thereof may not be reproduced in any form, stored in any retrieval system, or transmitted in any form by any means—electronic, mechanical, photocopy, recording, or otherwise—without prior written permission of the Publisher

Color Test Page

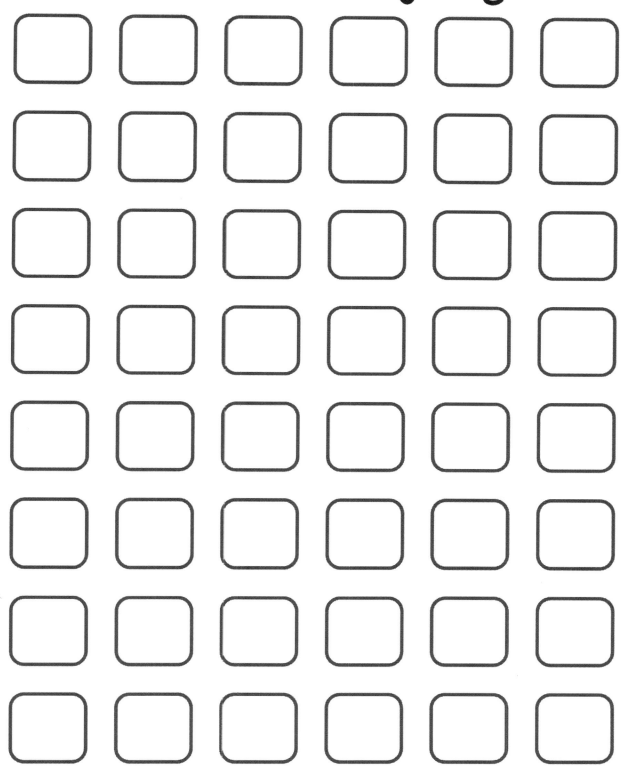

Color Test Page

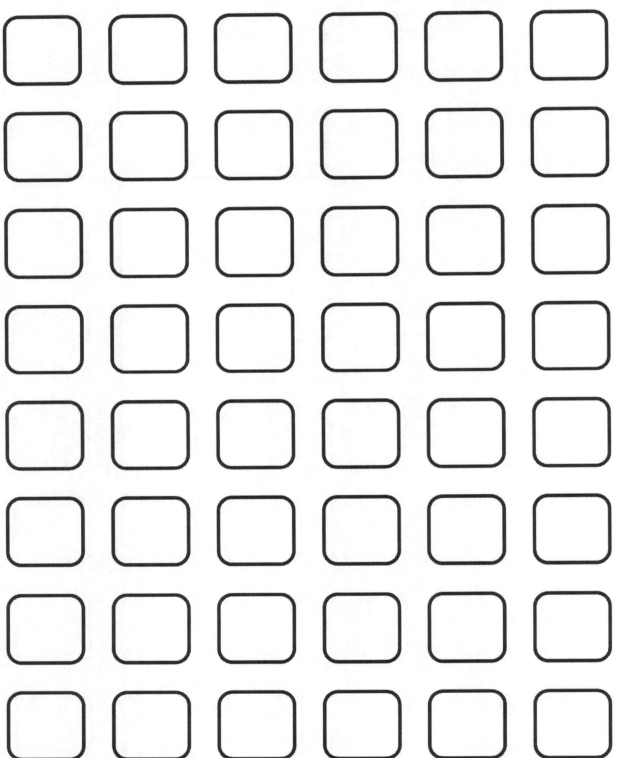

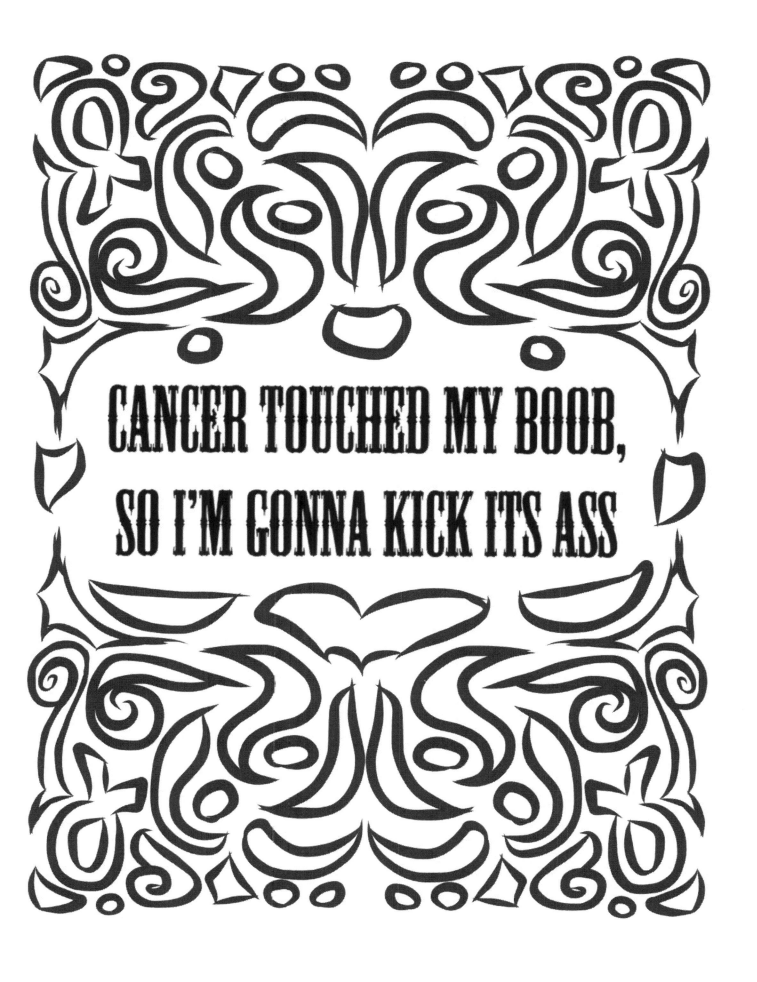

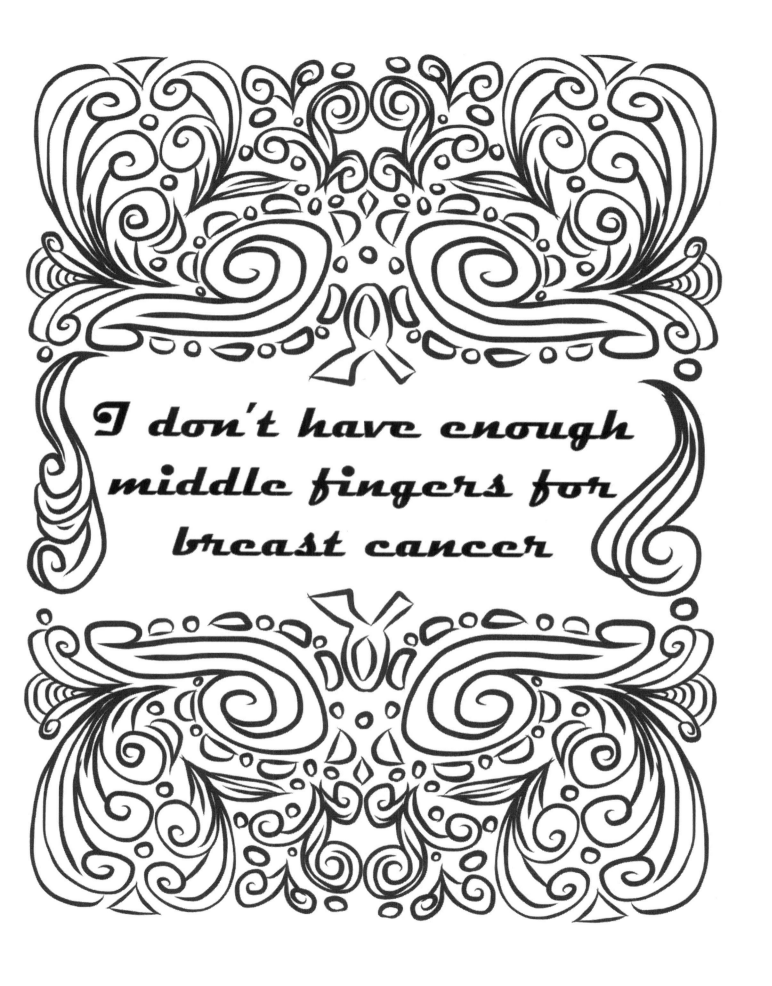

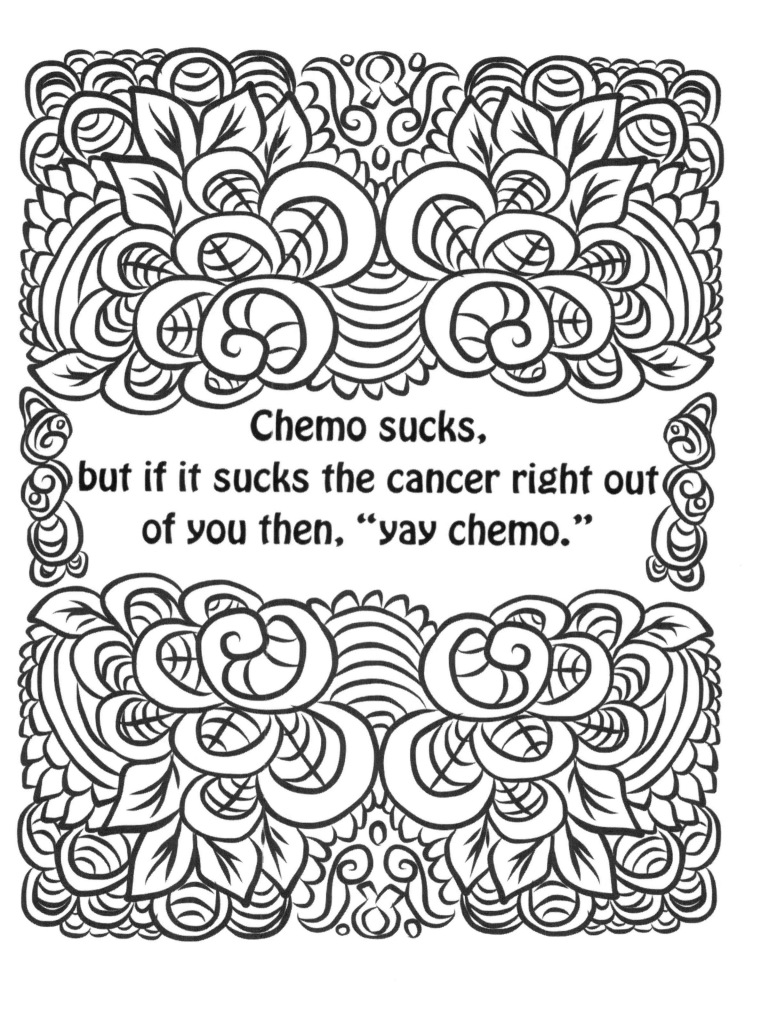

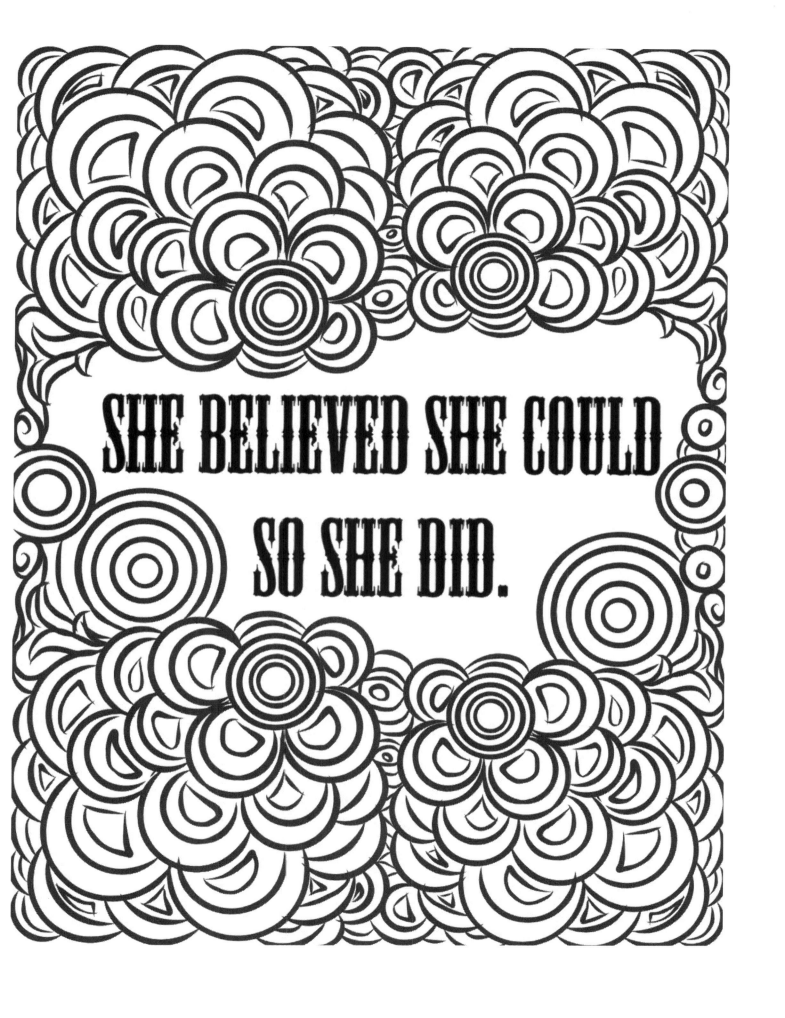

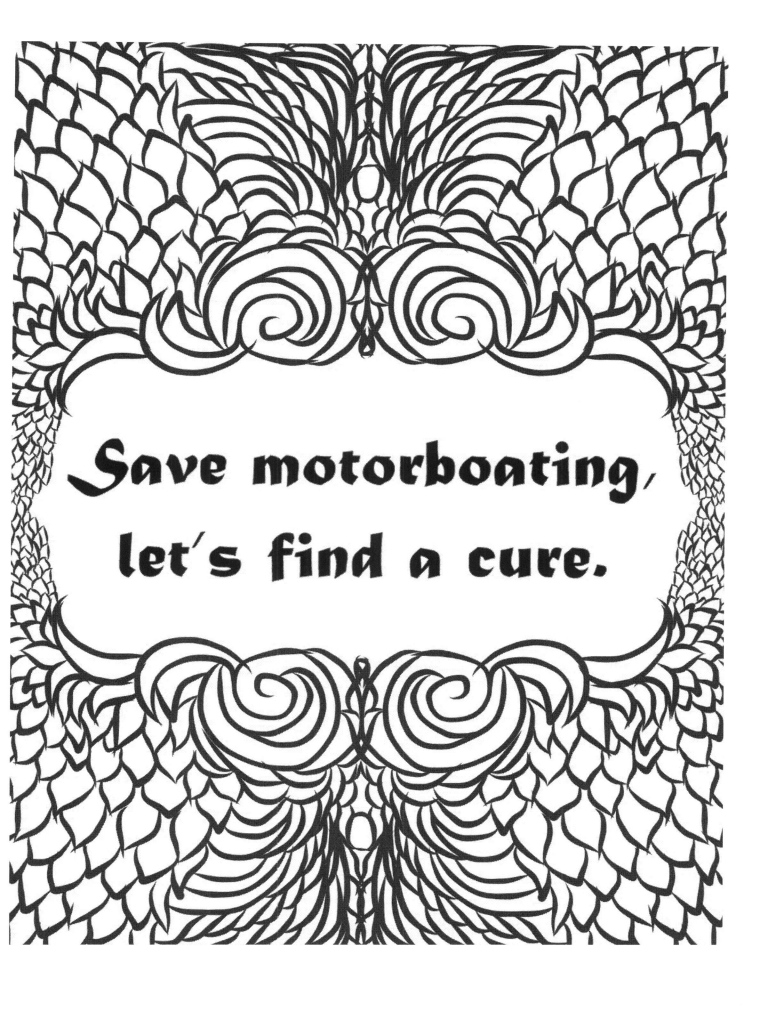

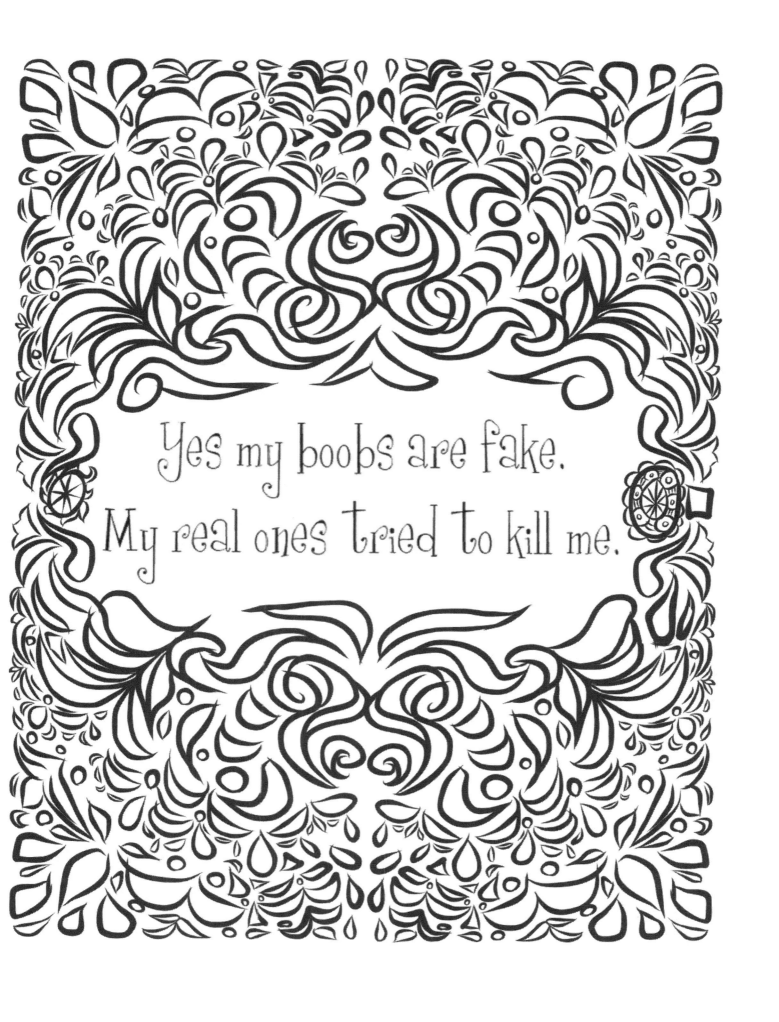

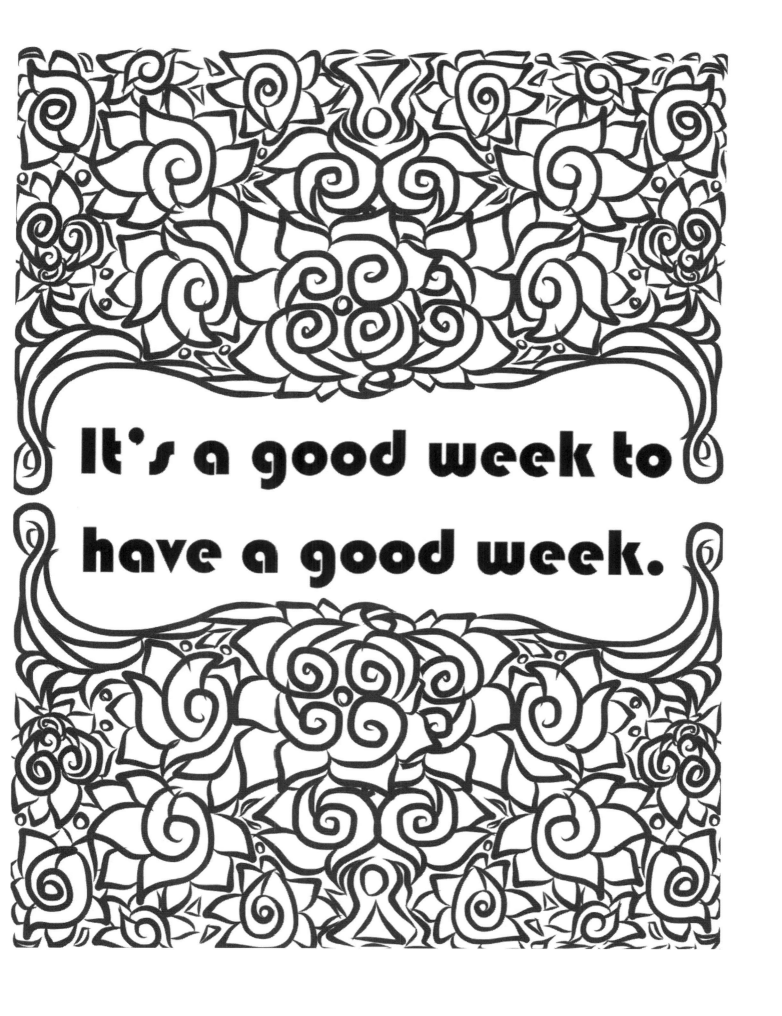

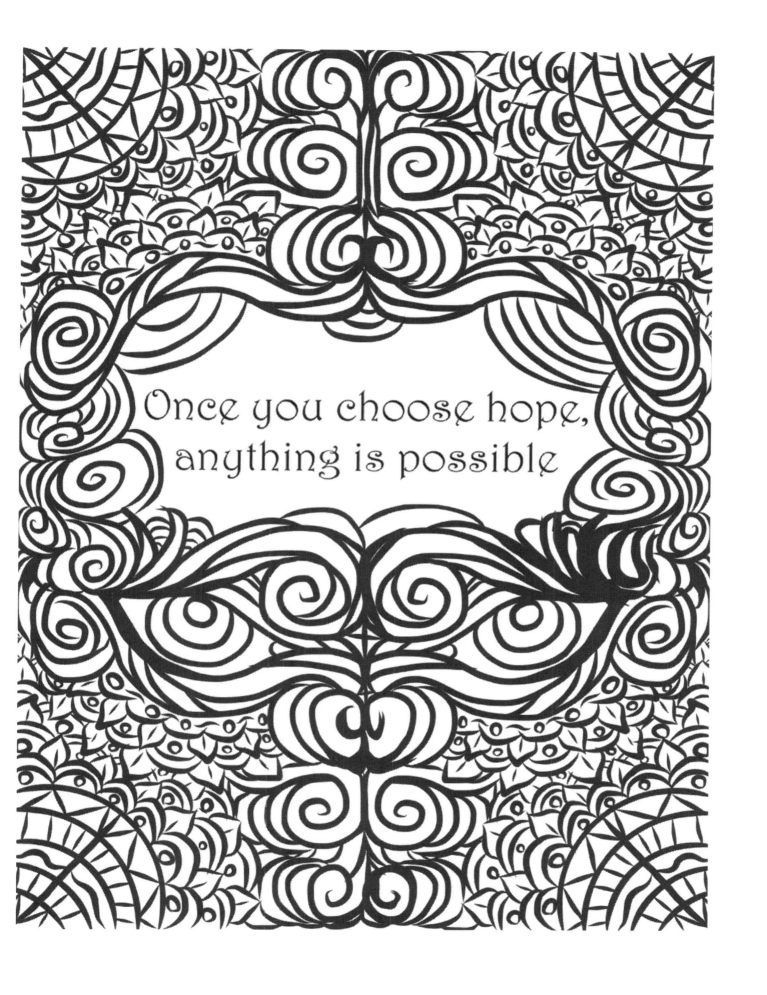

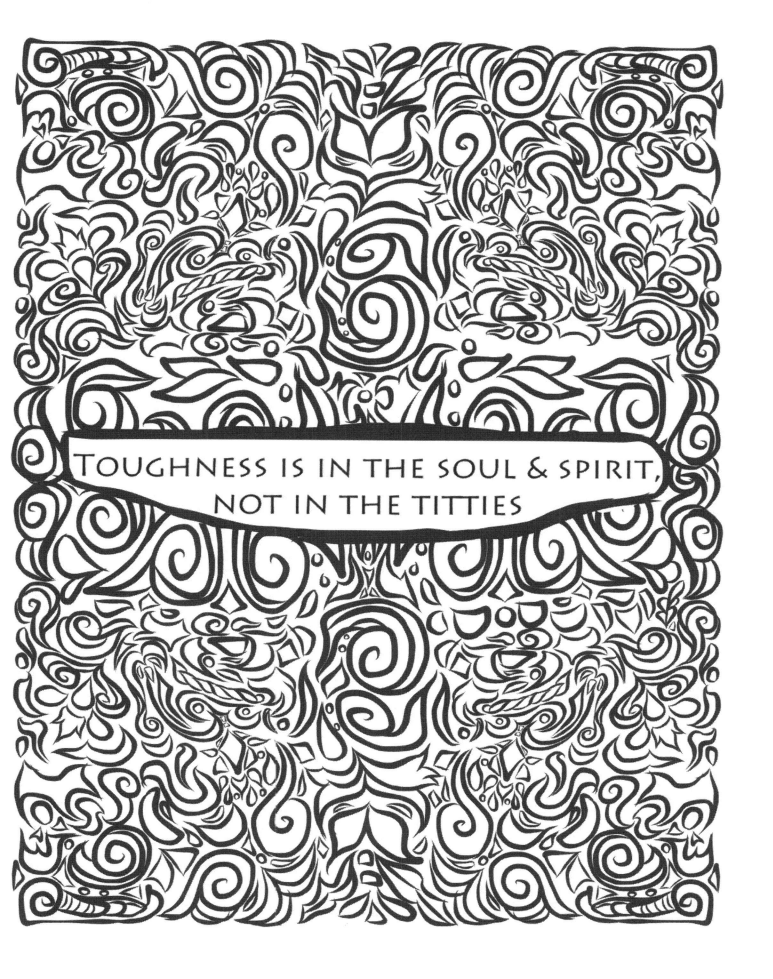

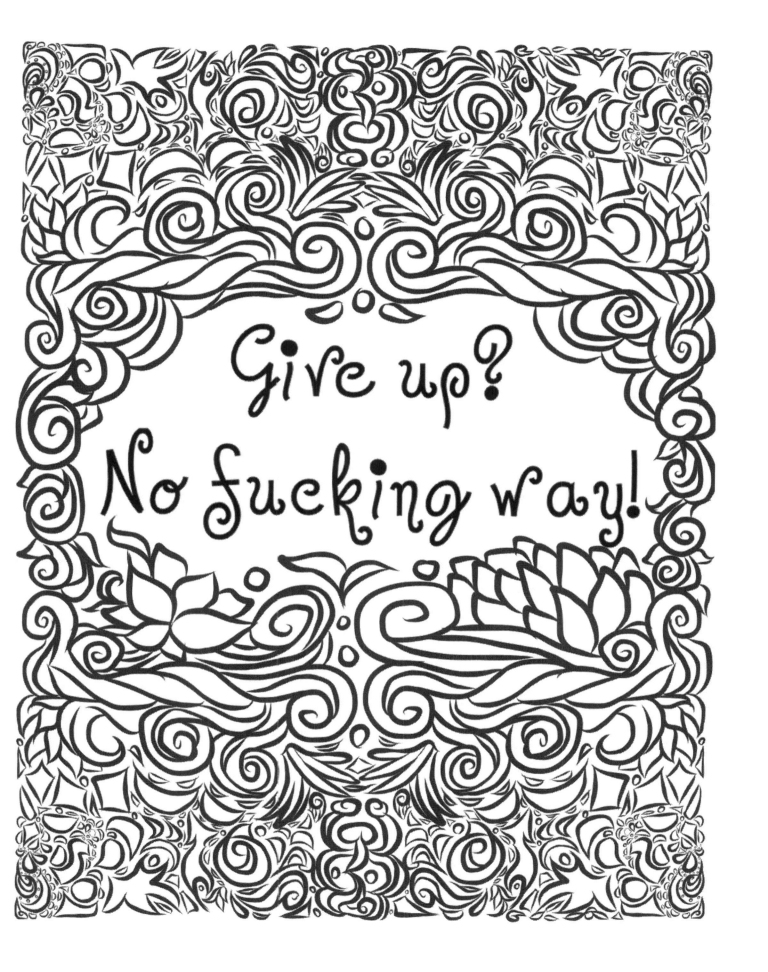

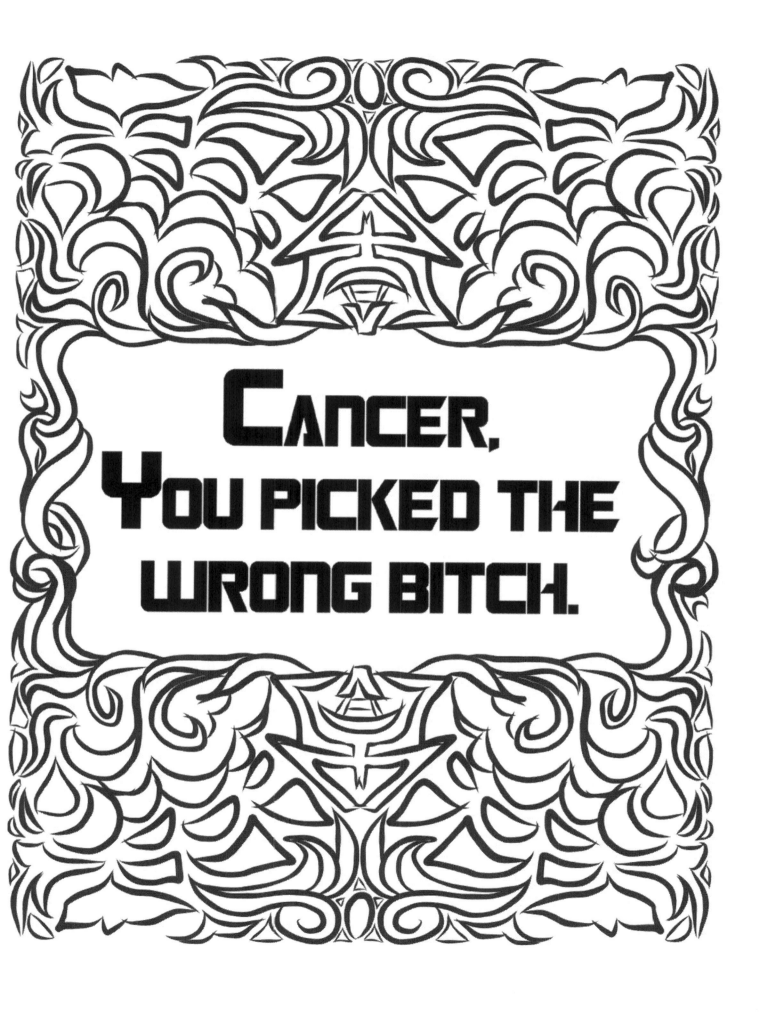

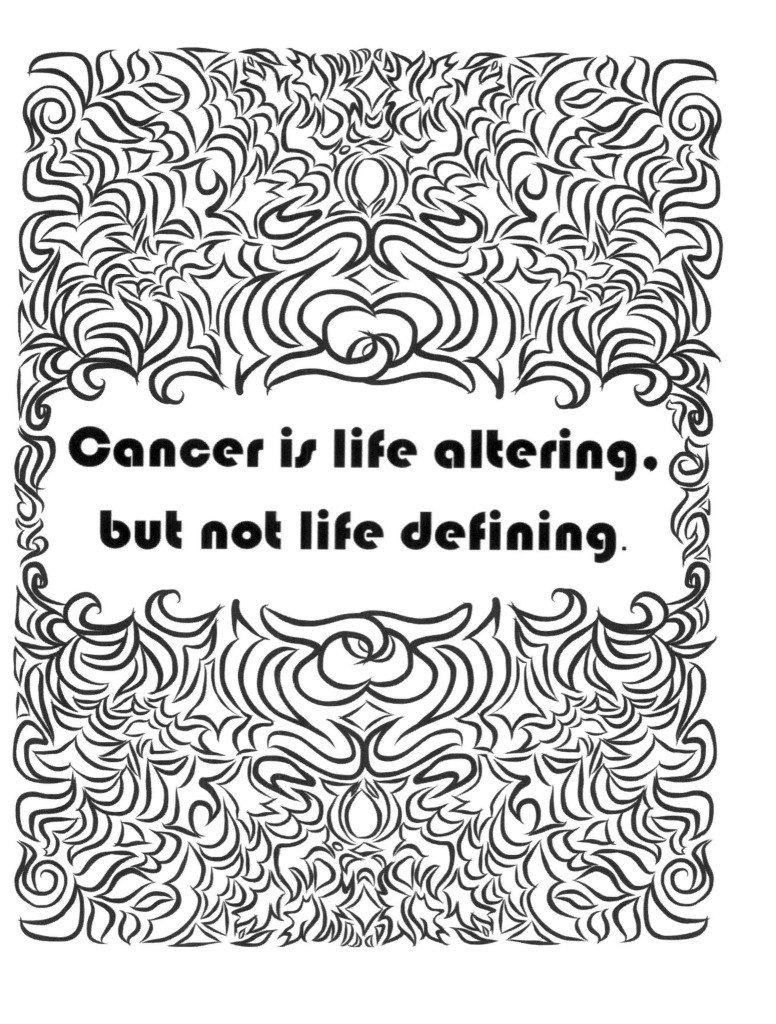

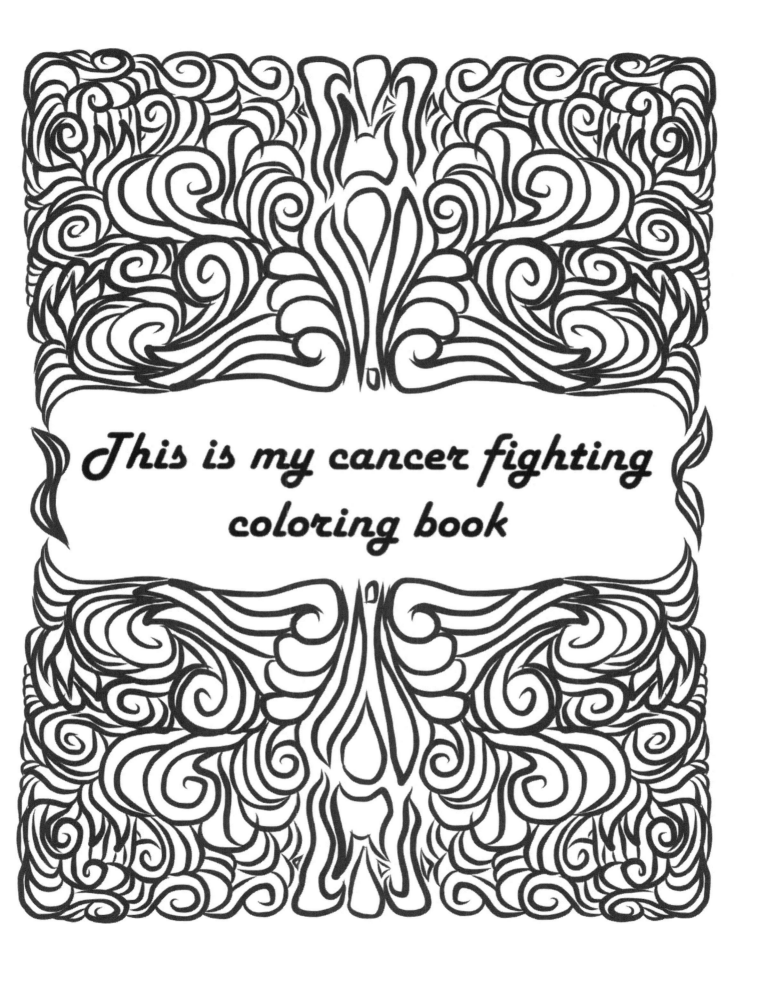

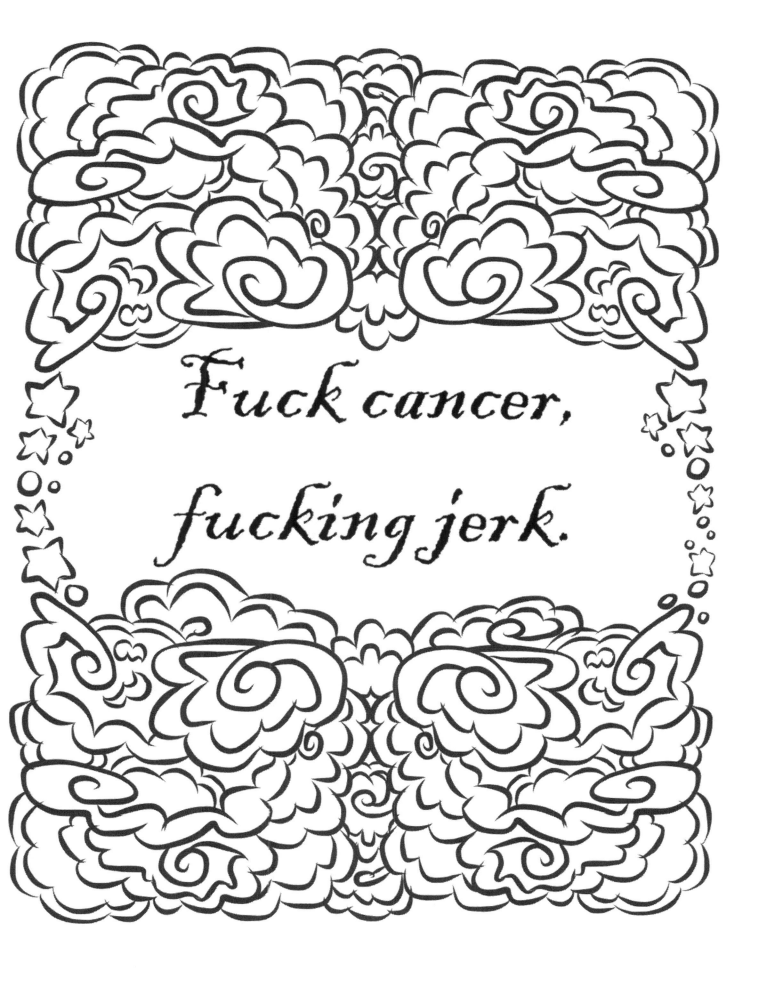

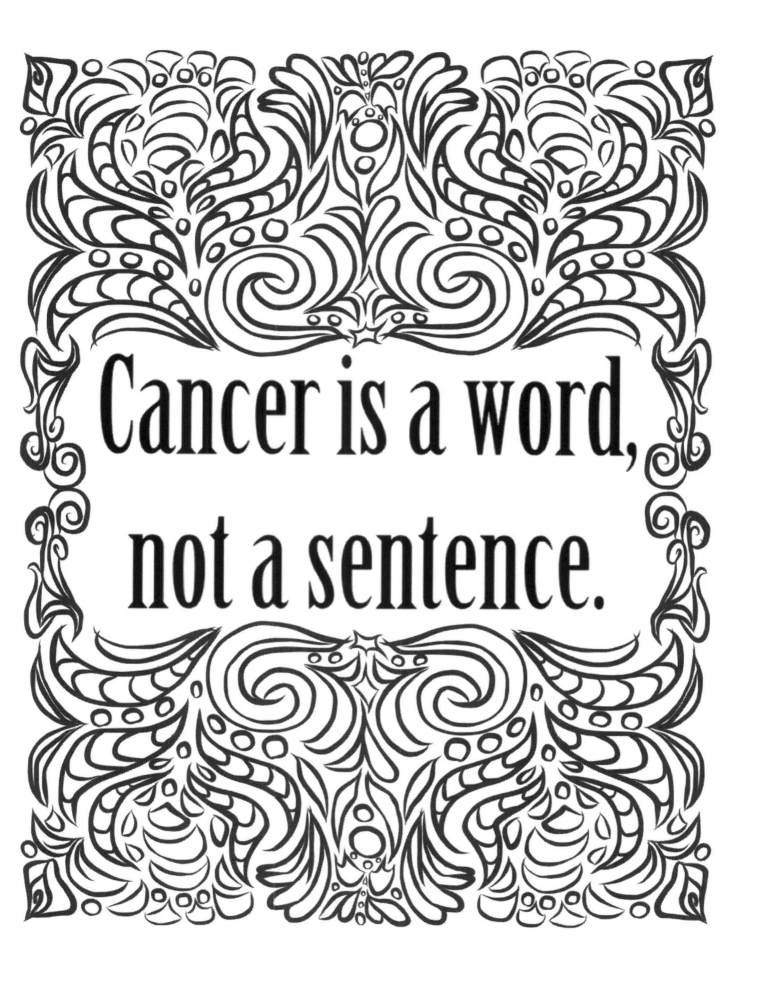

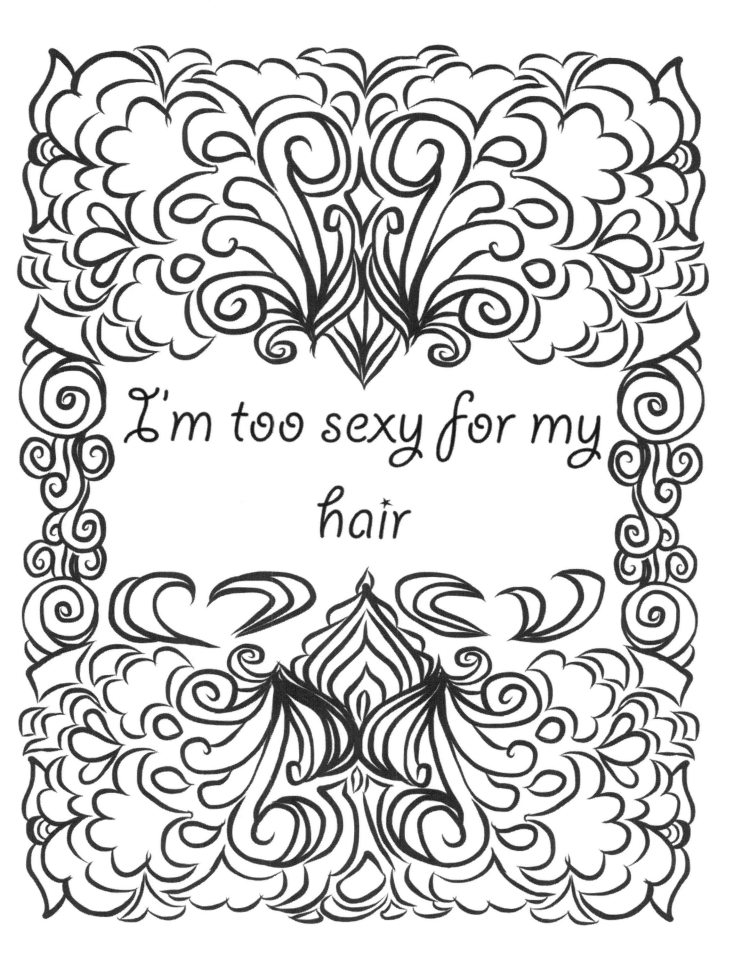

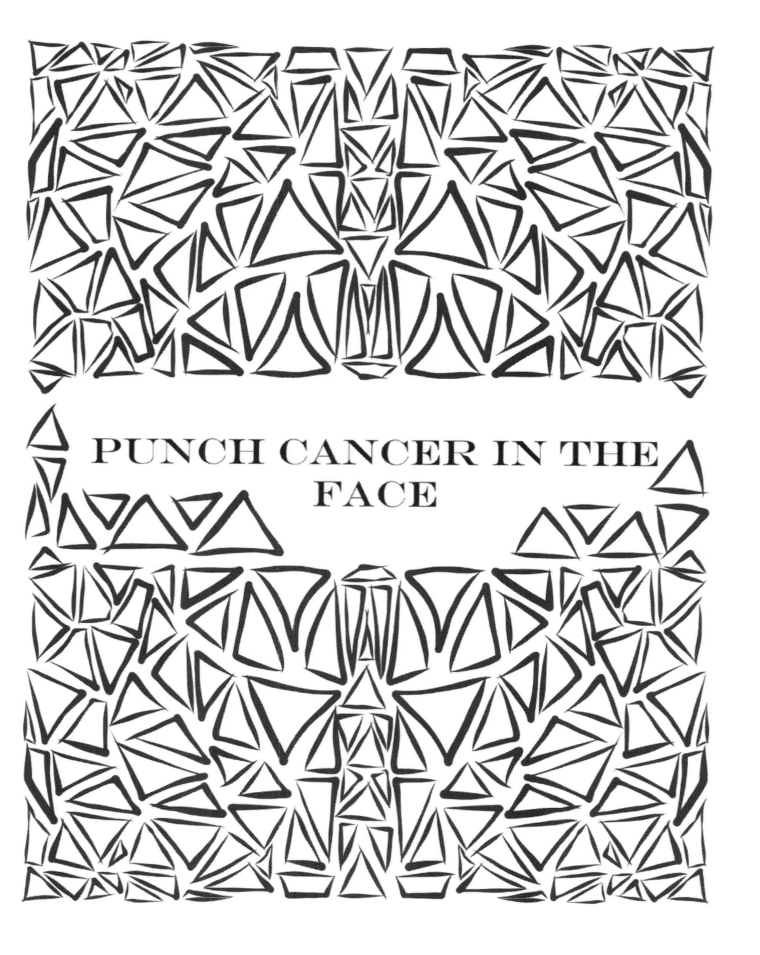

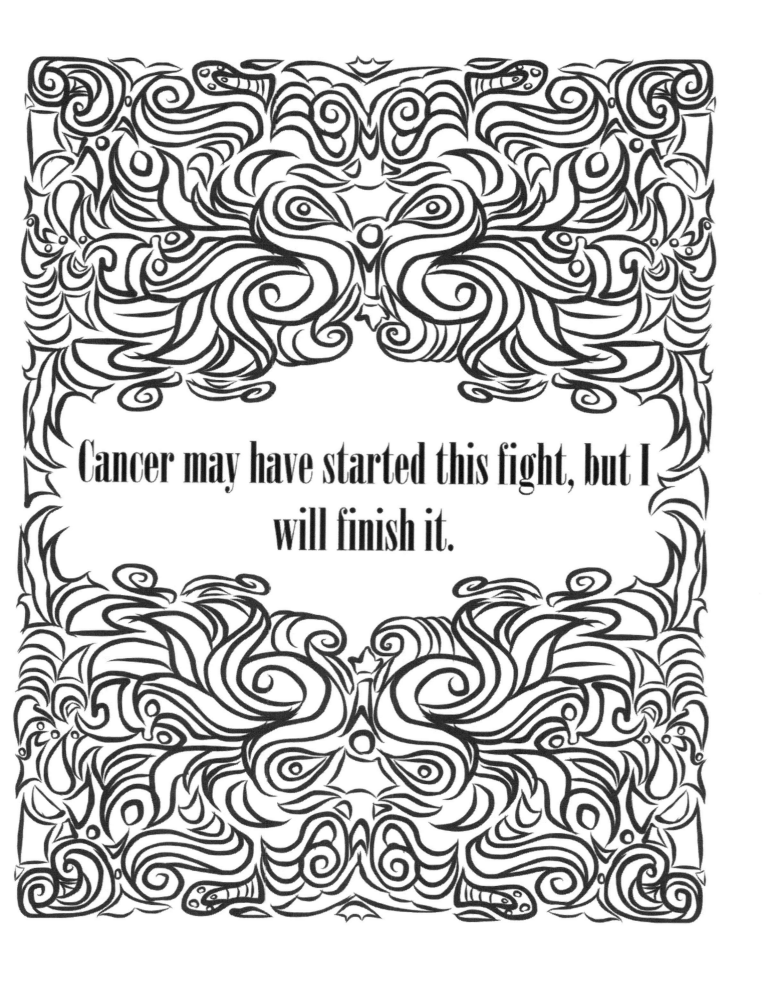

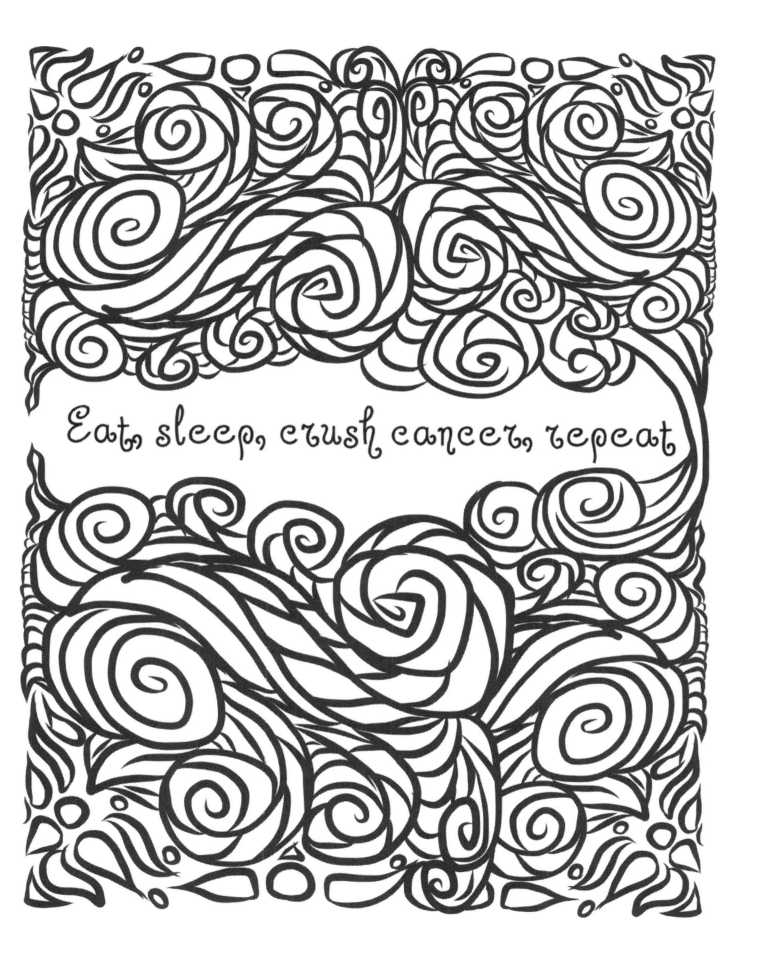

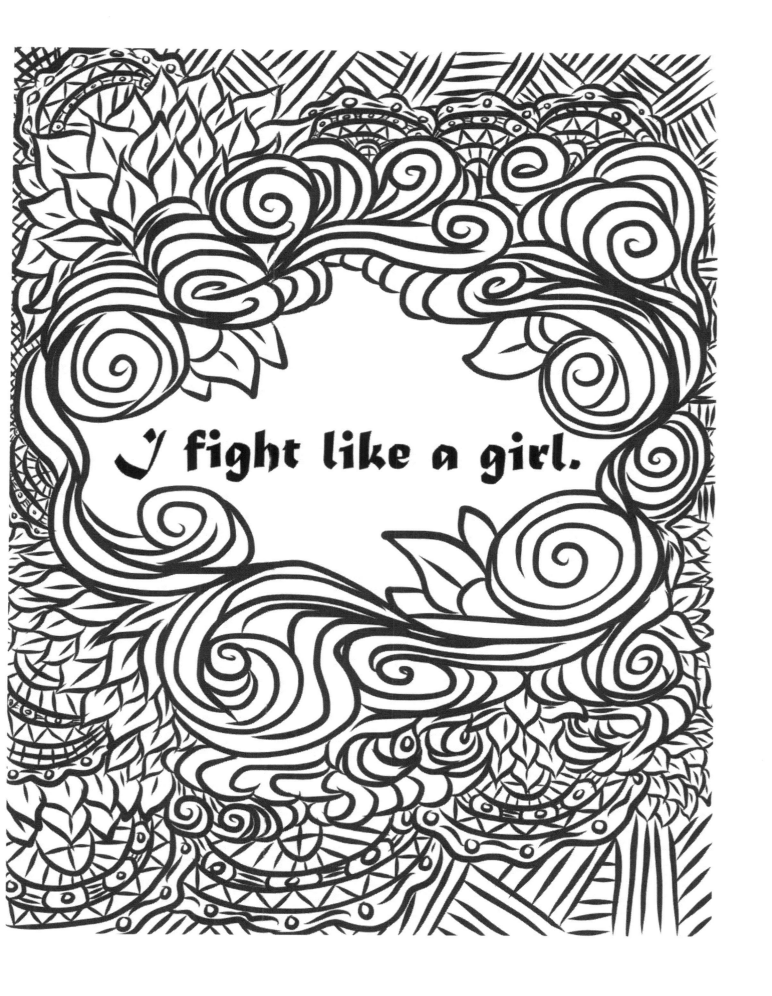

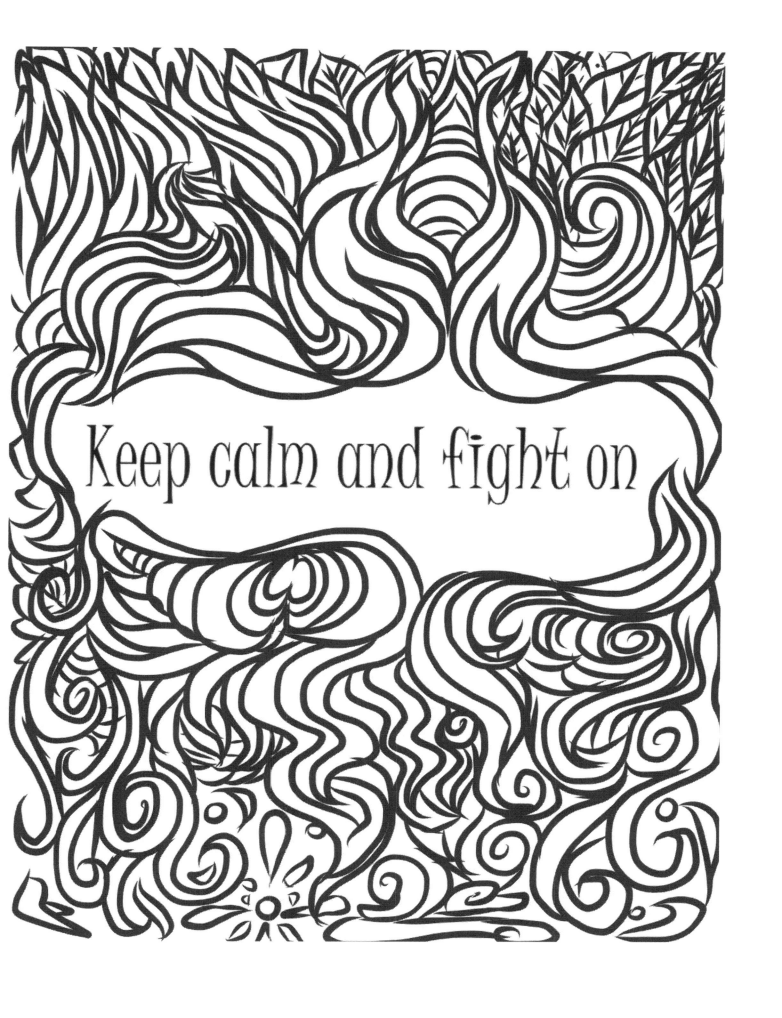

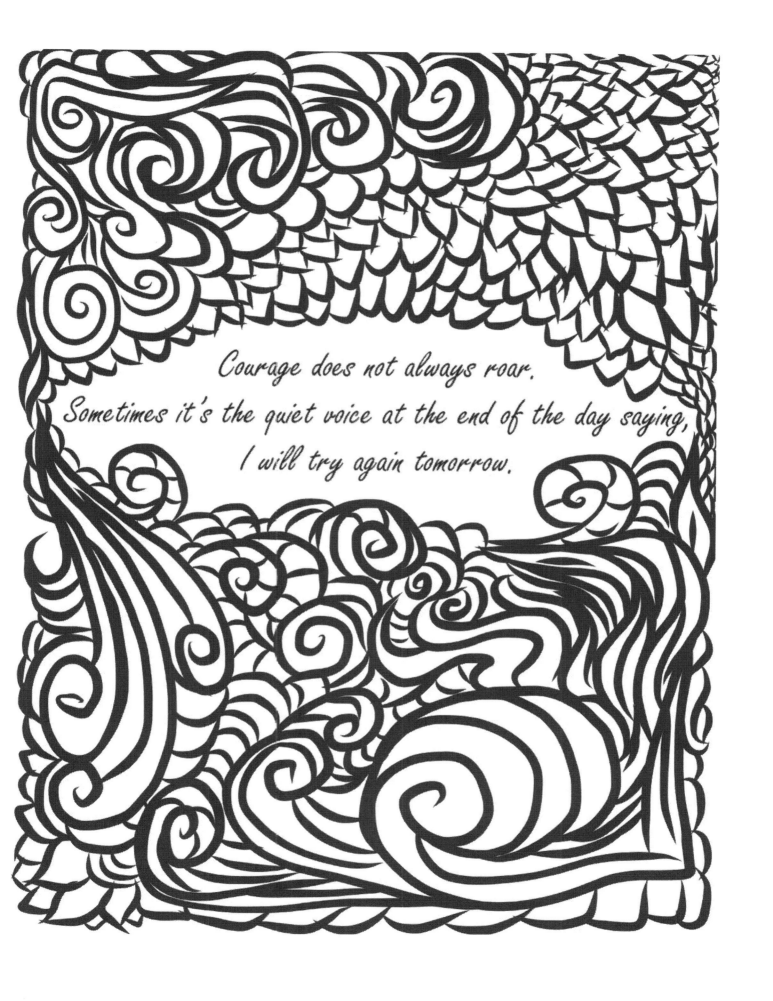

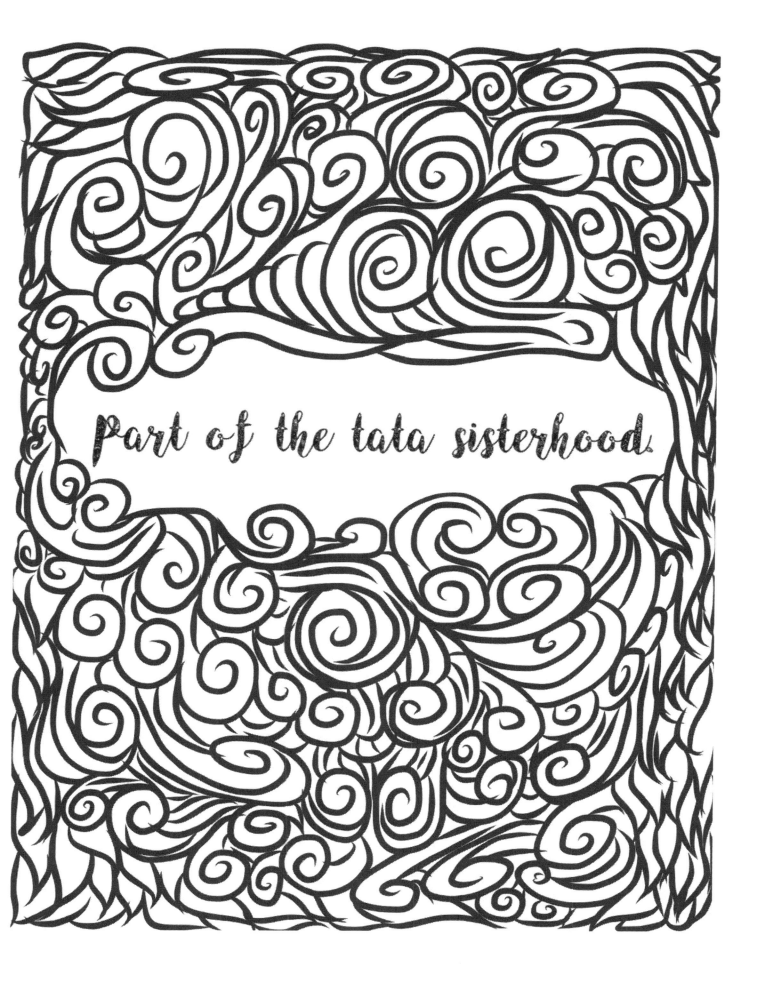

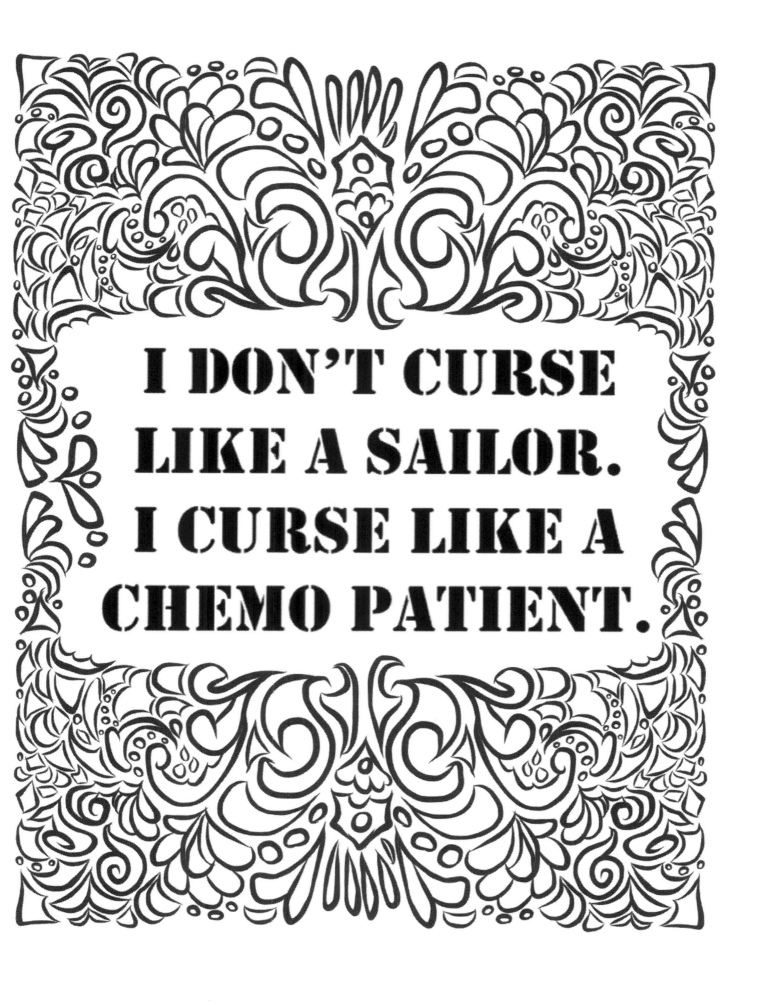

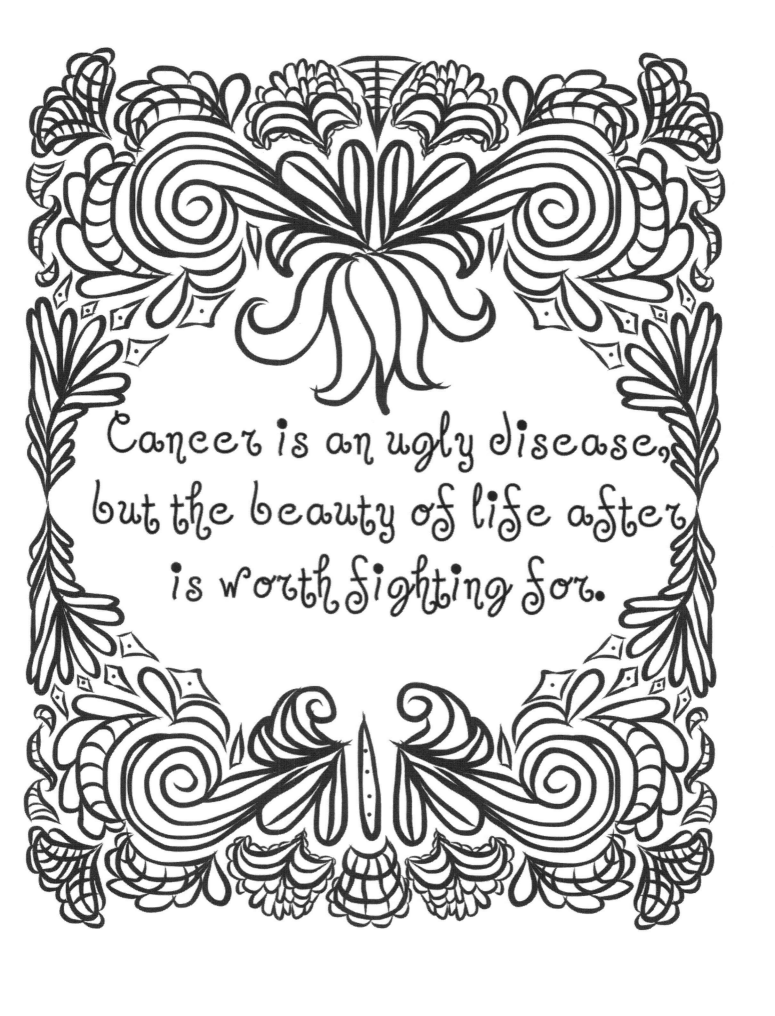

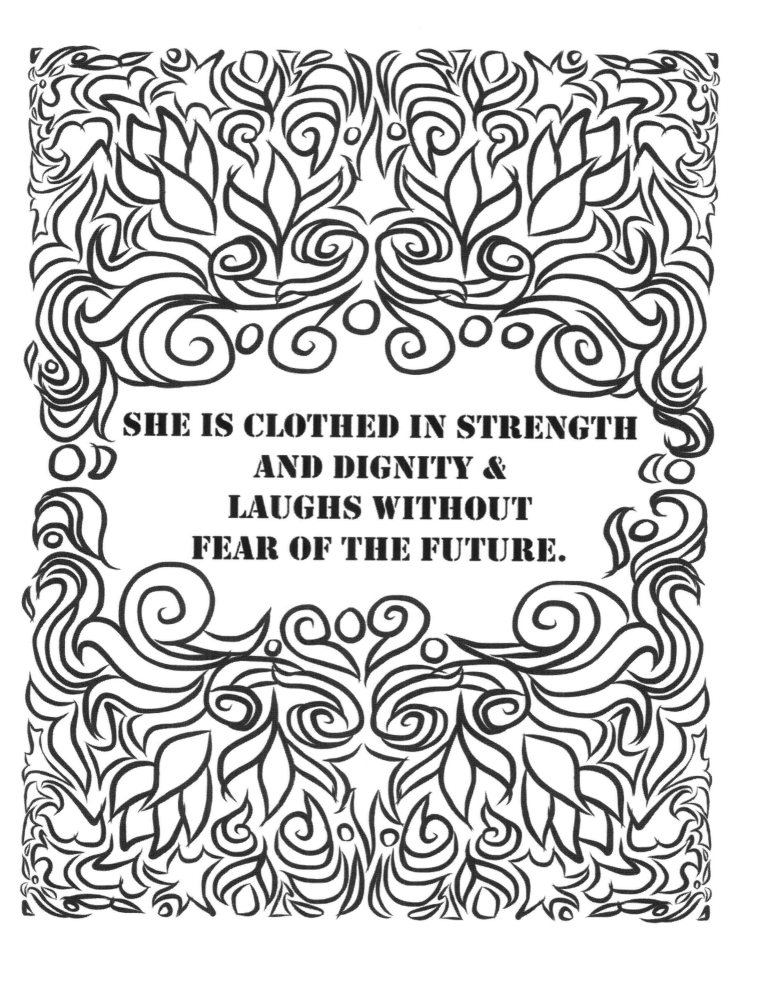

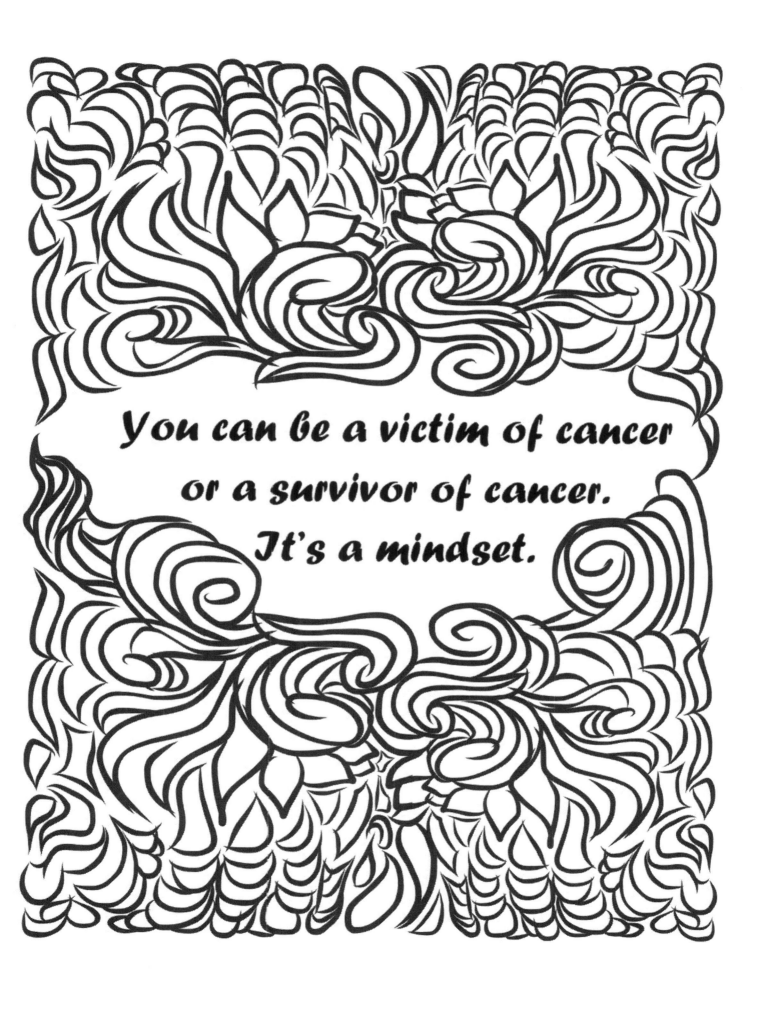

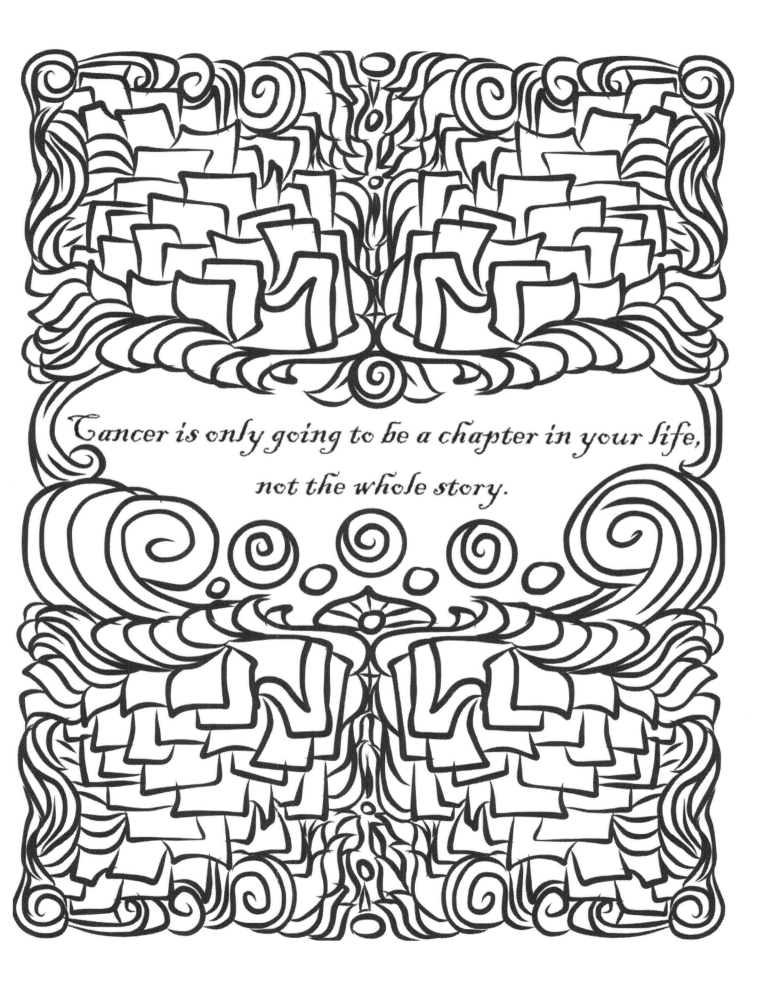

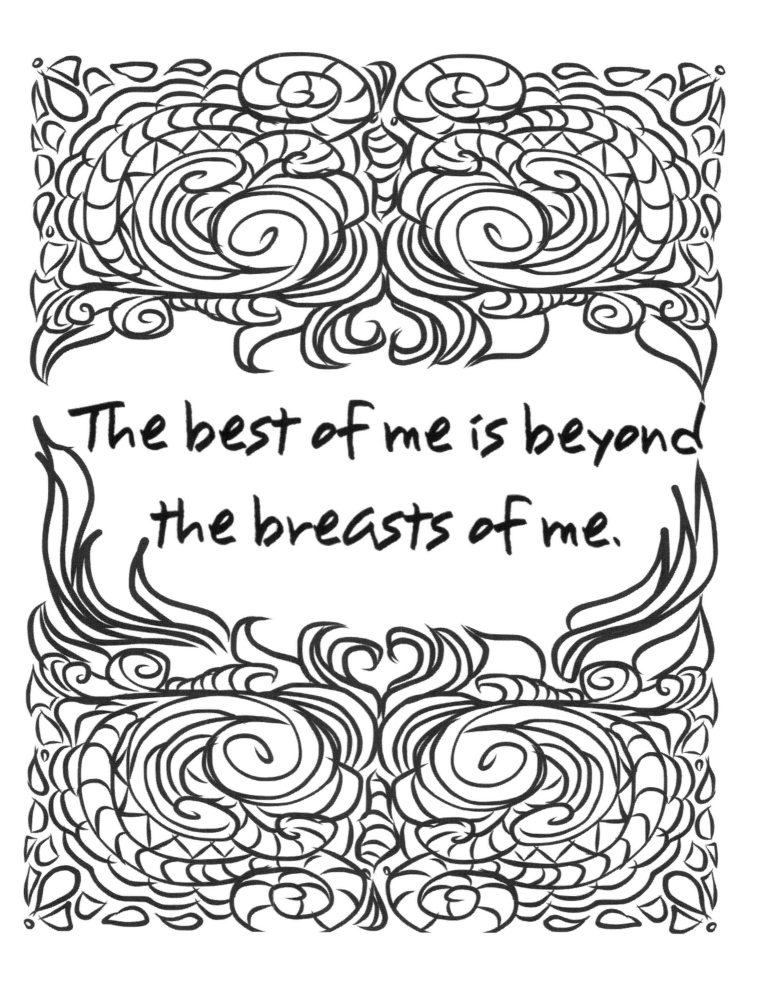

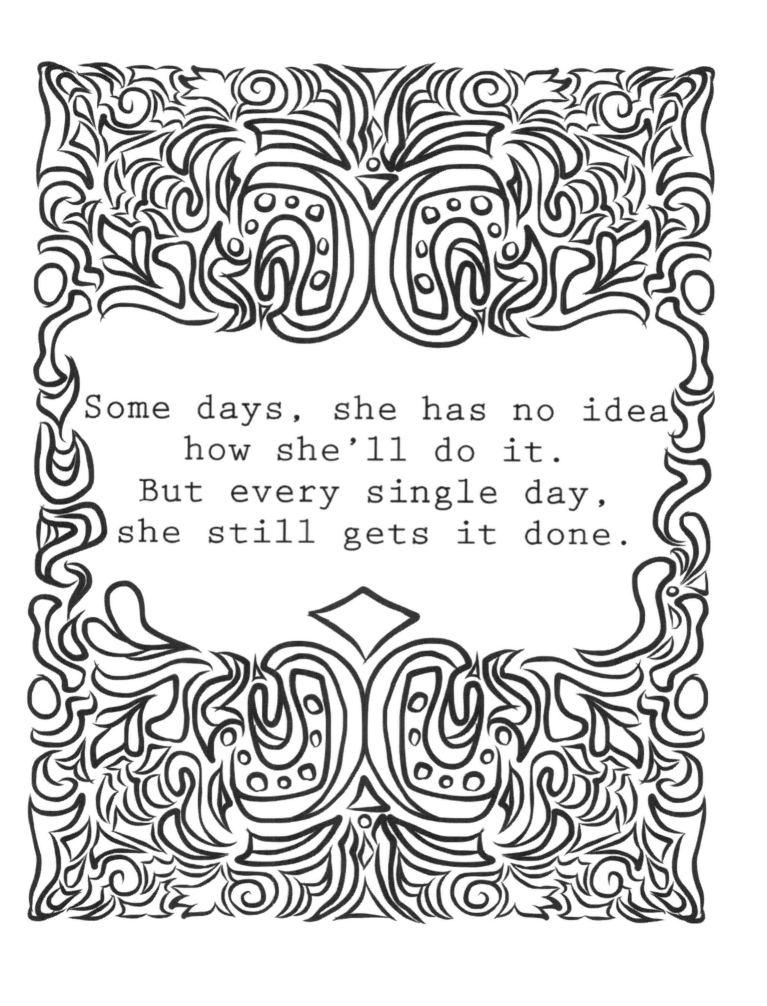

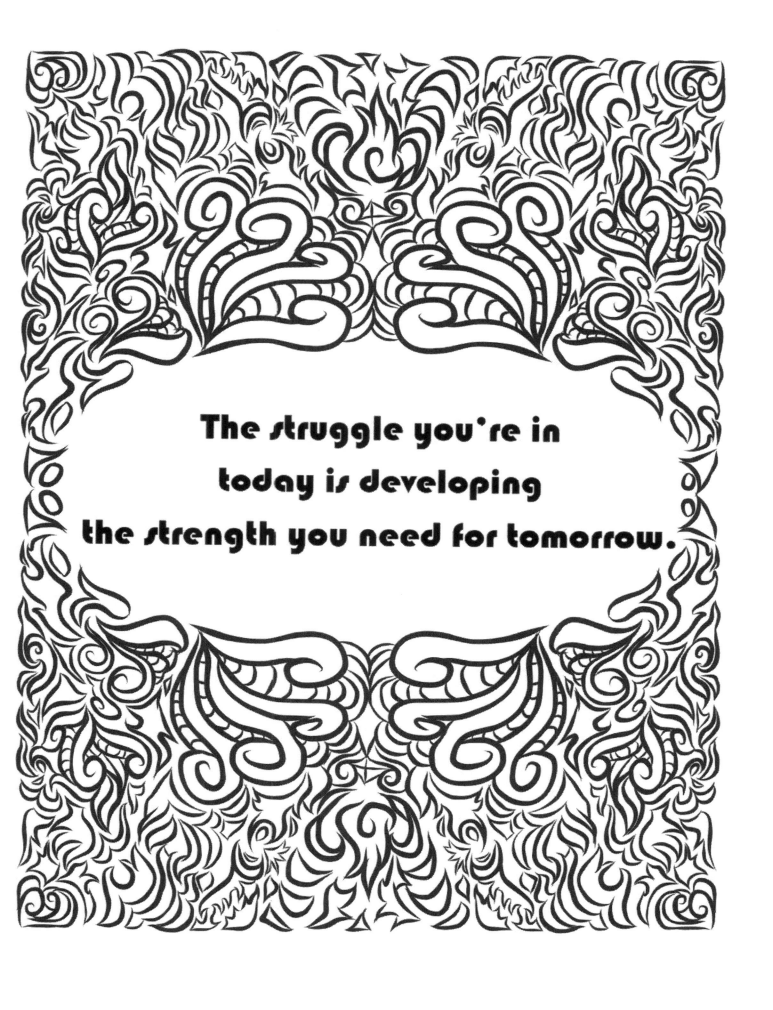

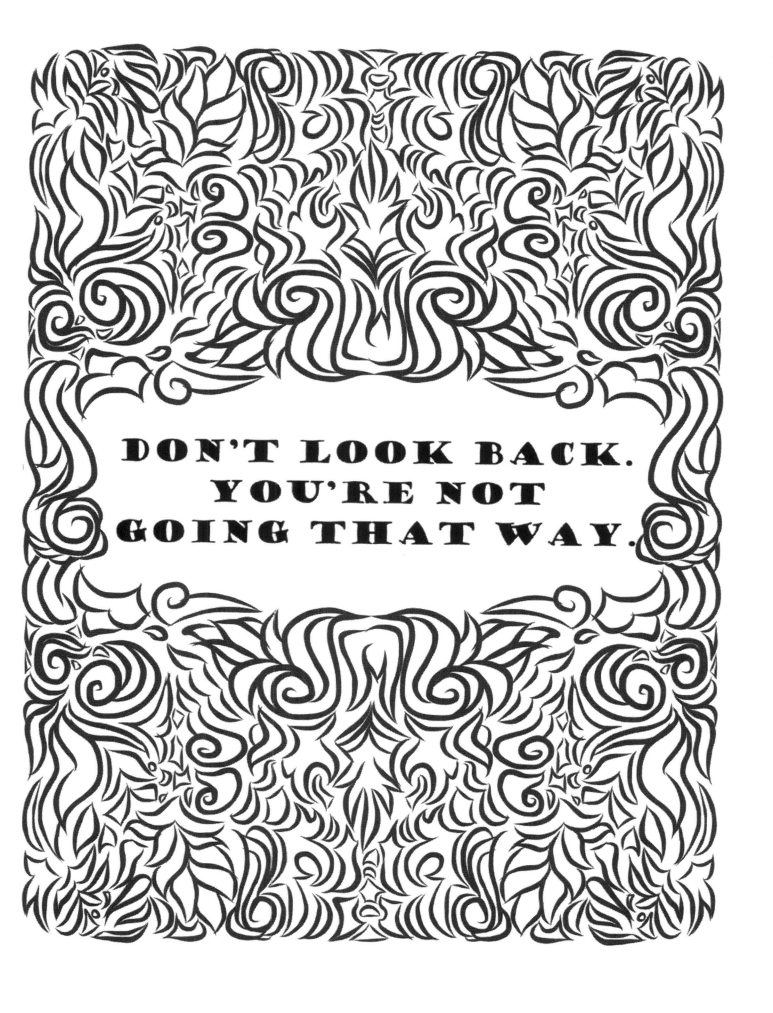

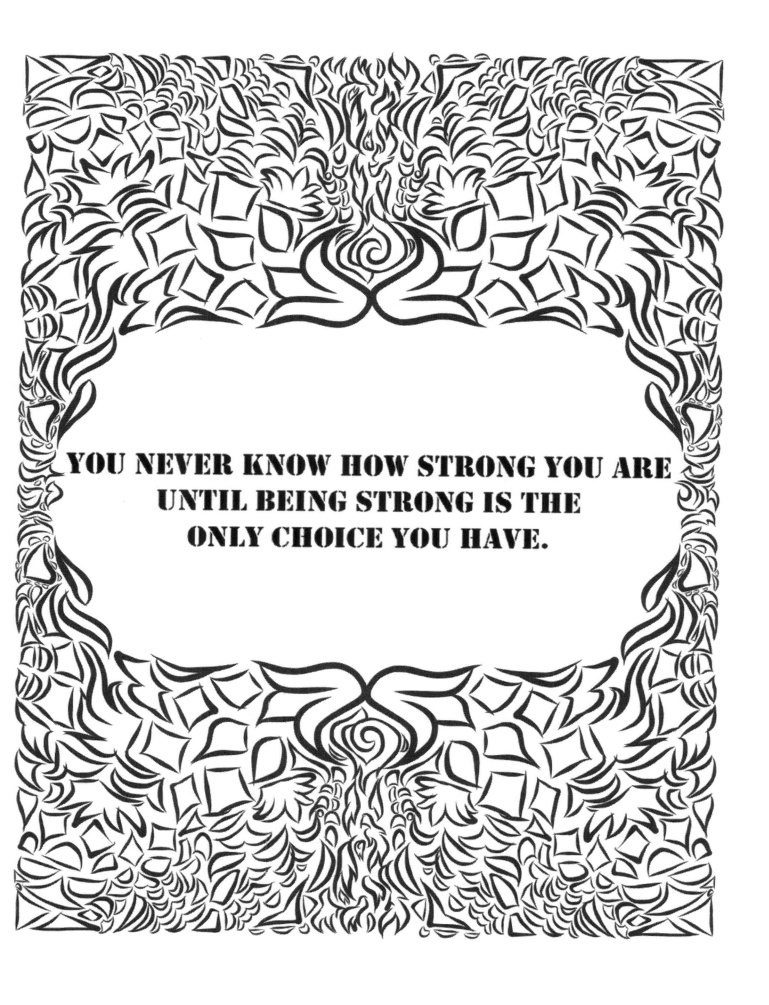

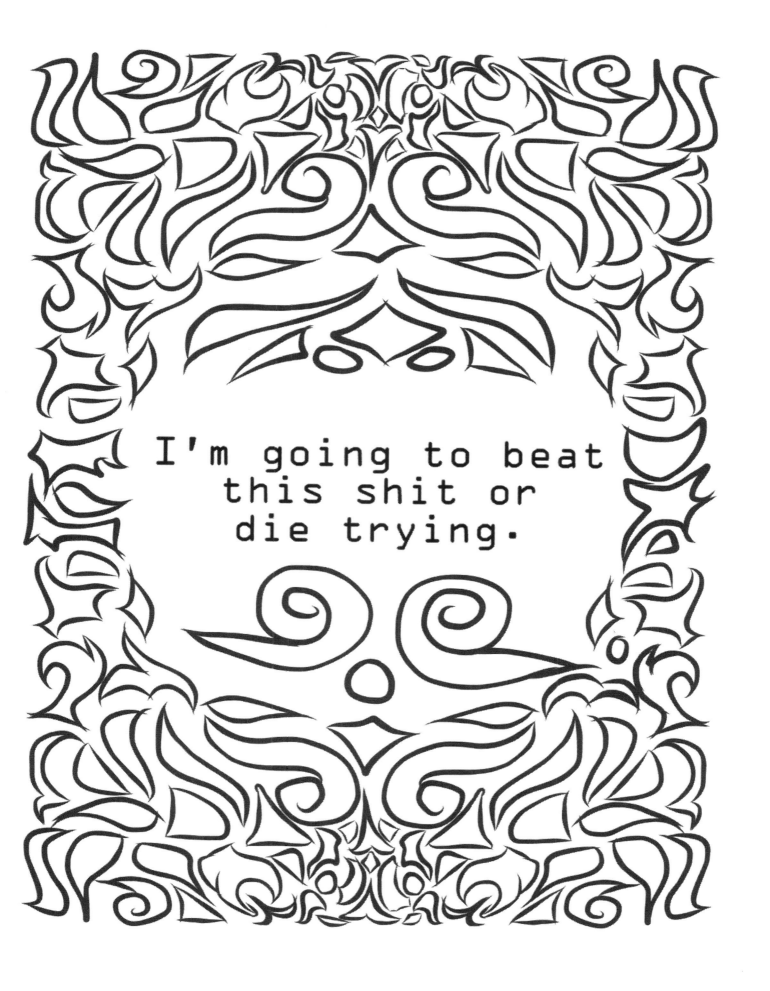

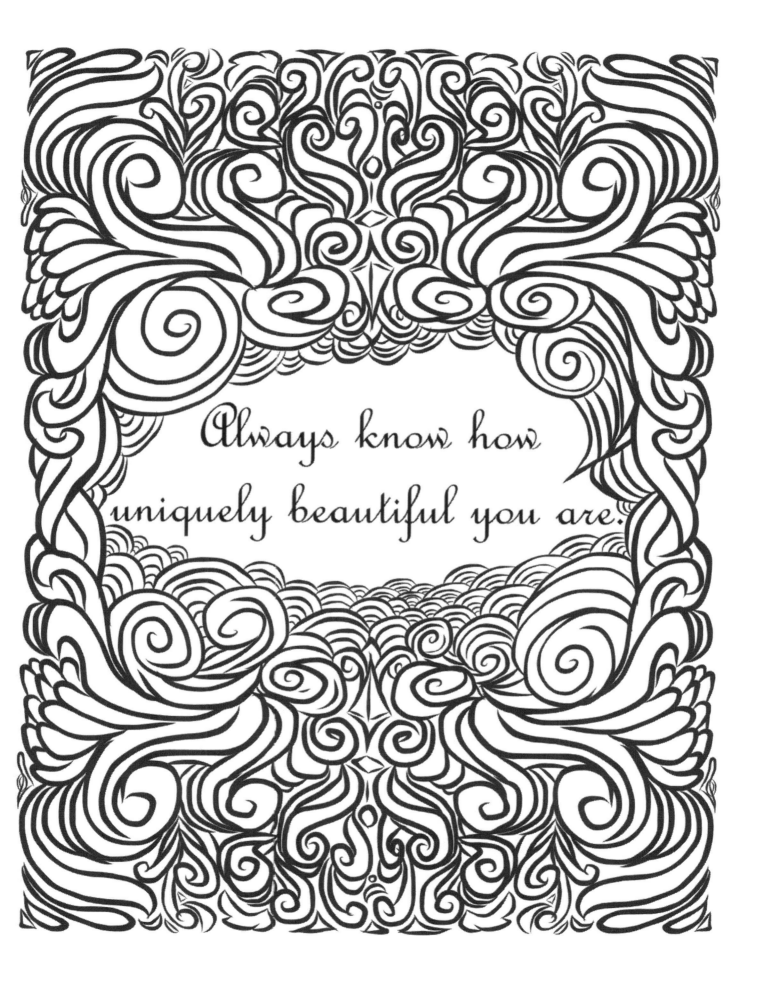

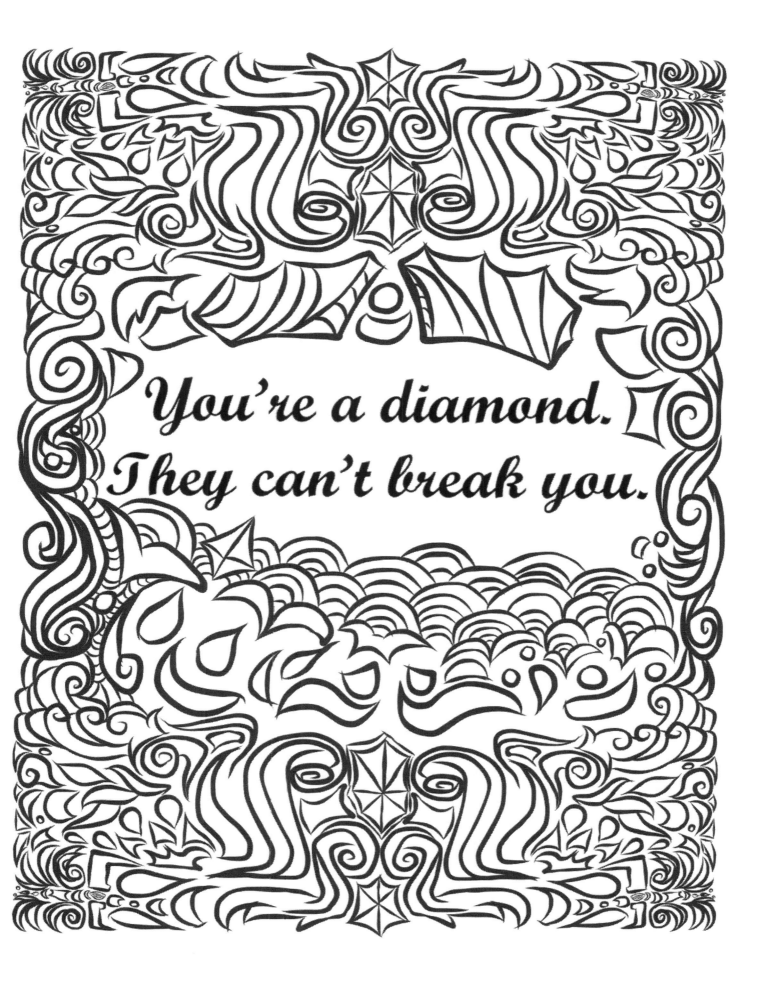

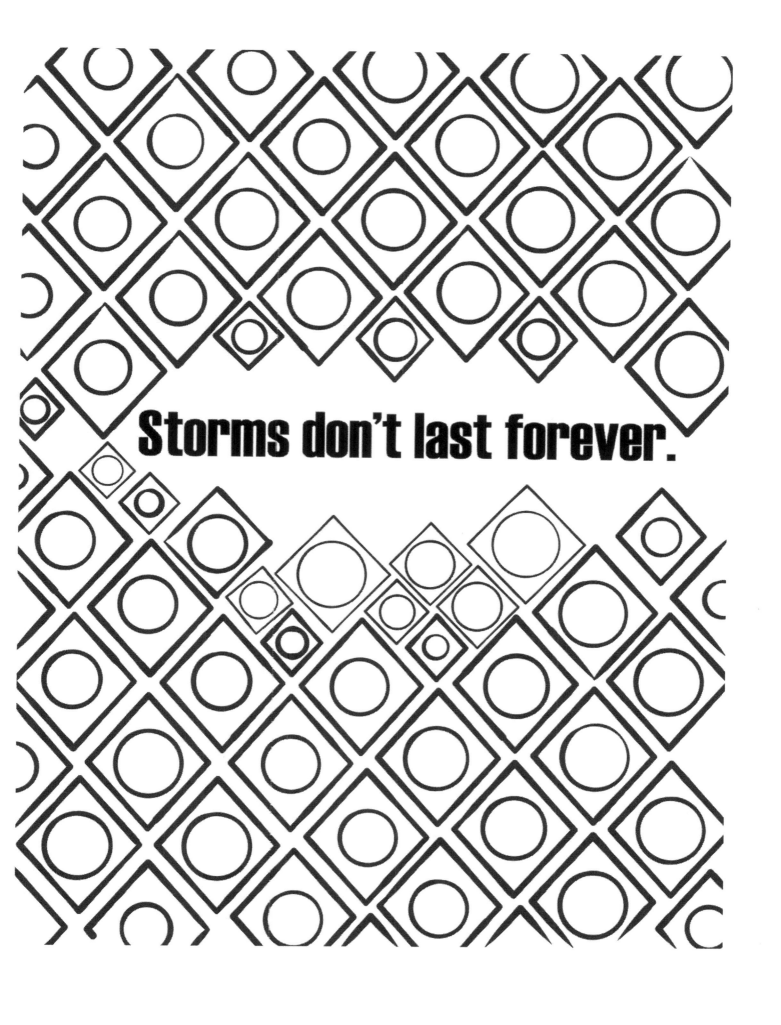

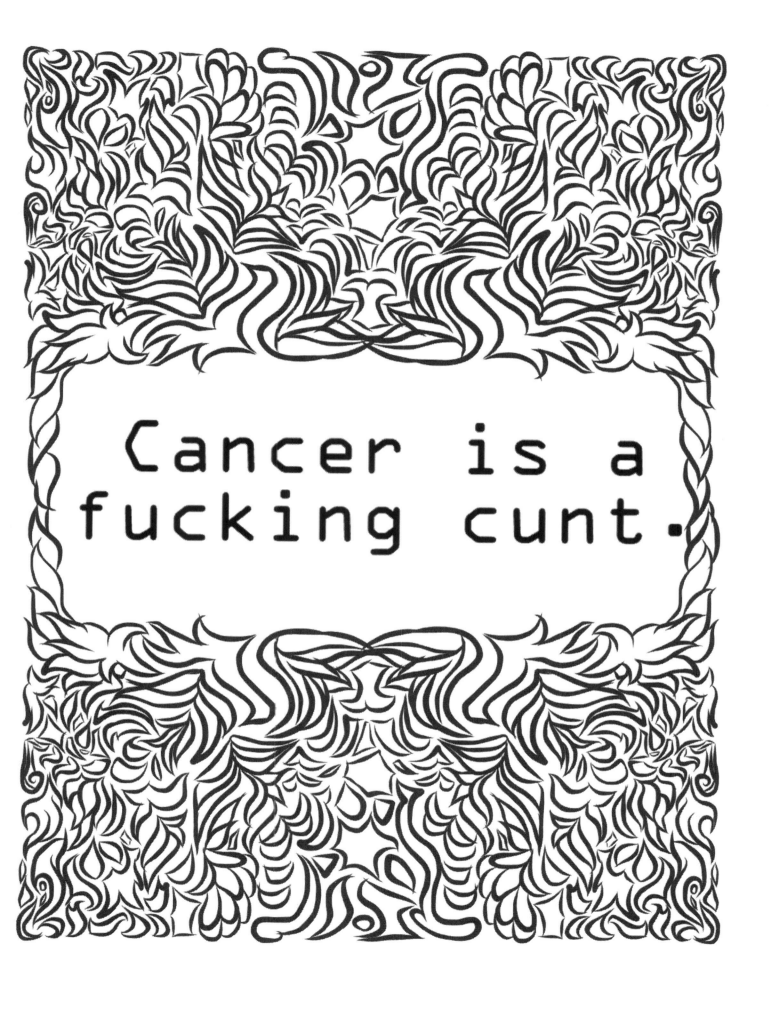

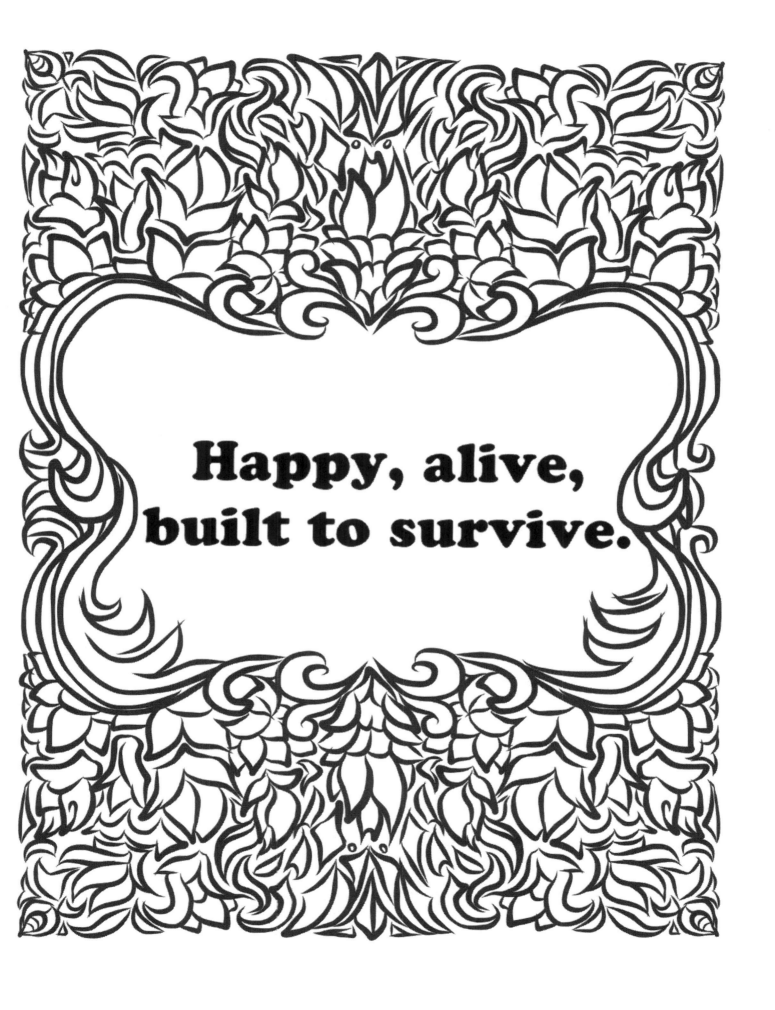

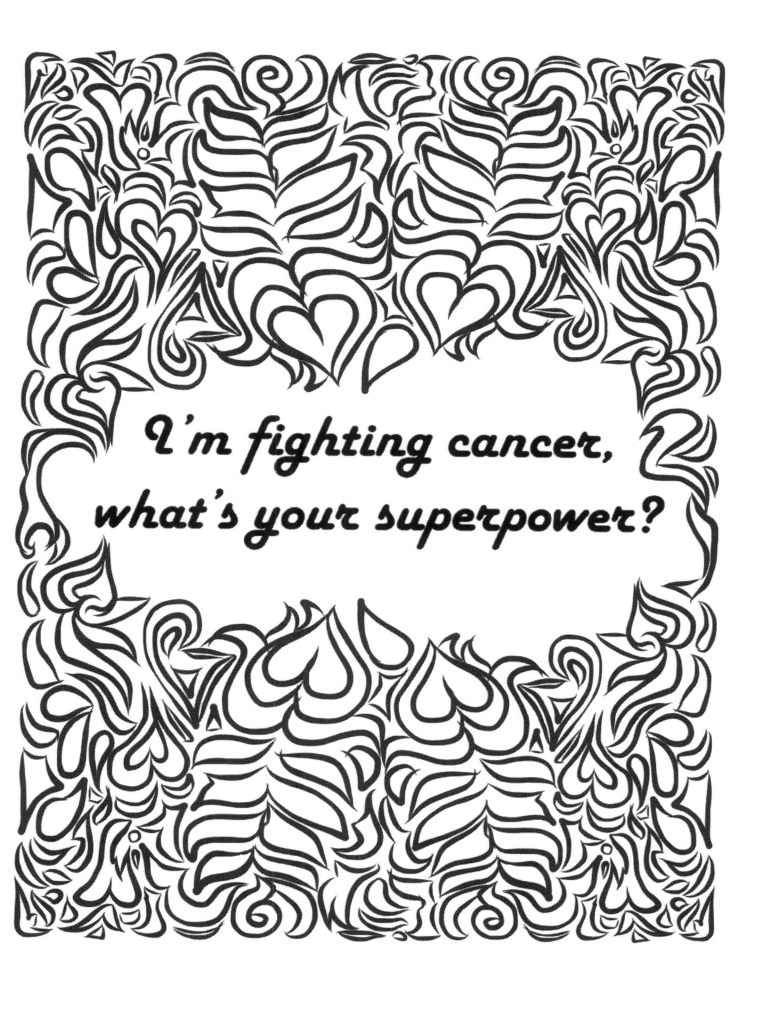

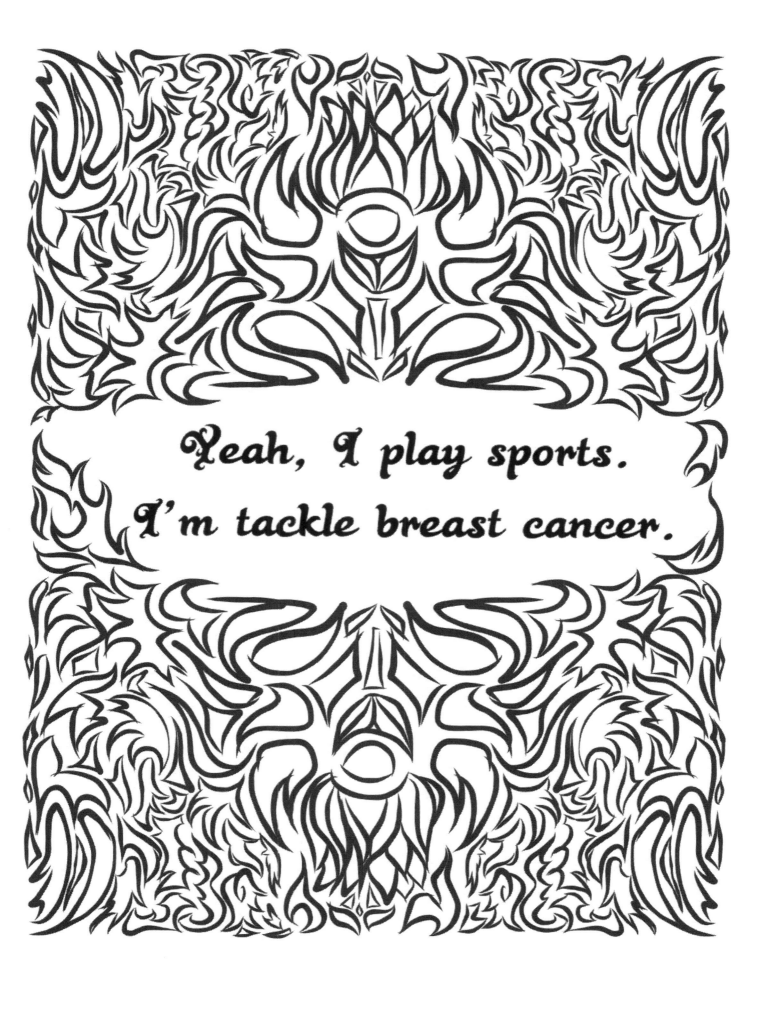

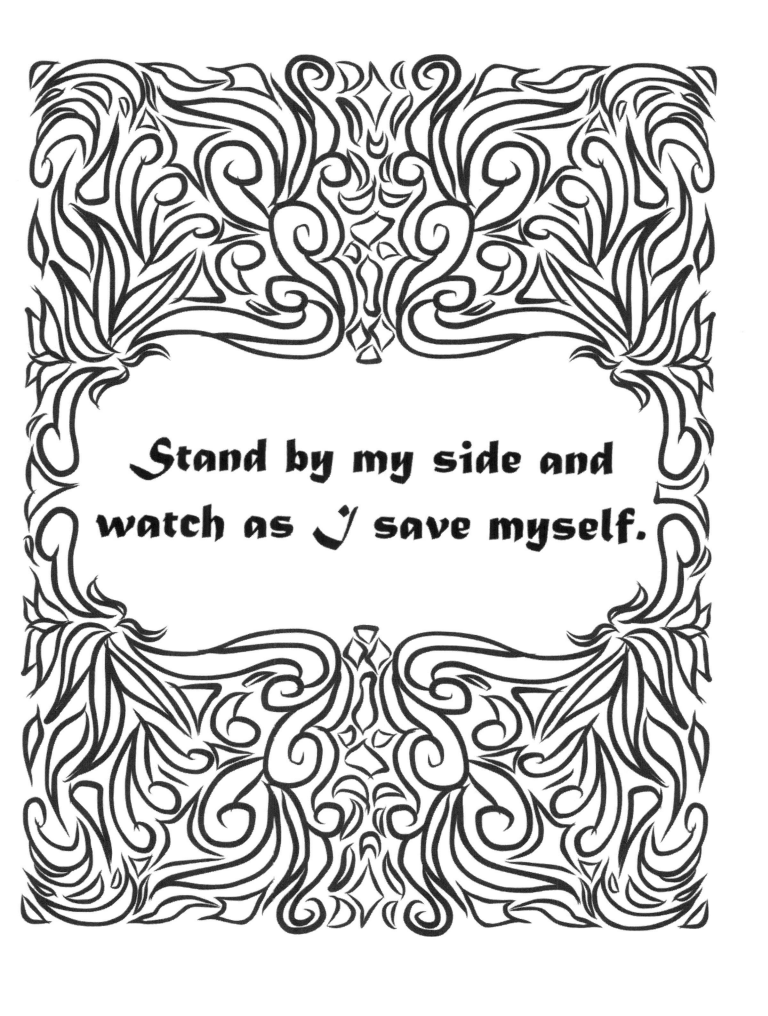

Stand by my side and watch as I save myself.

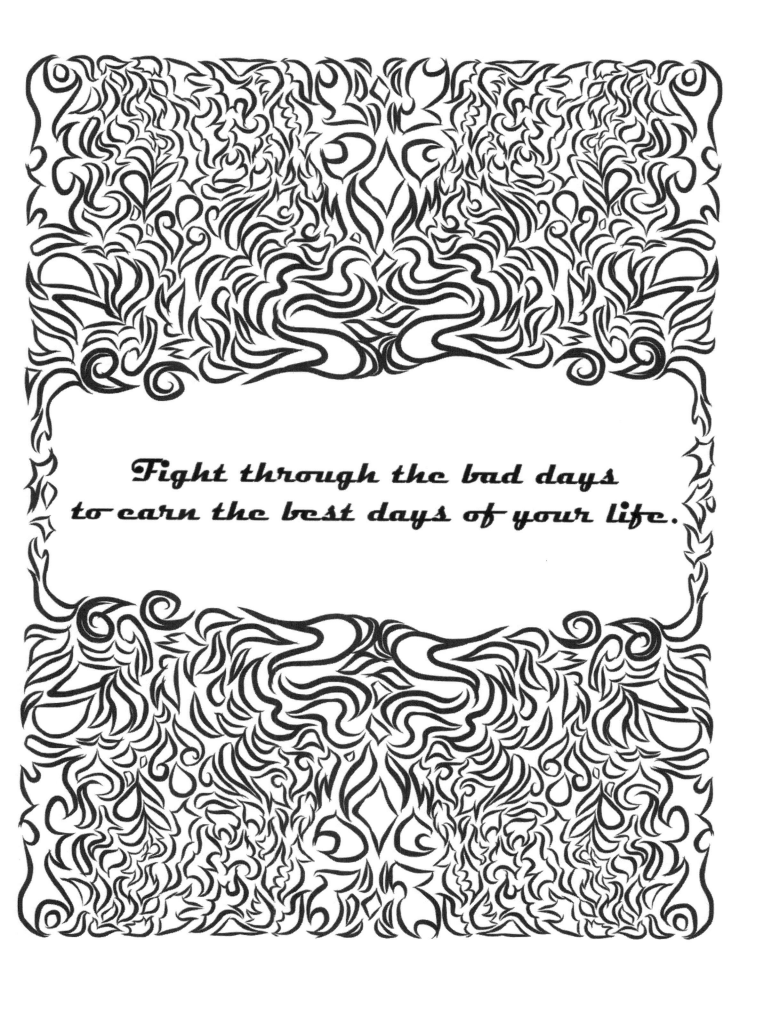

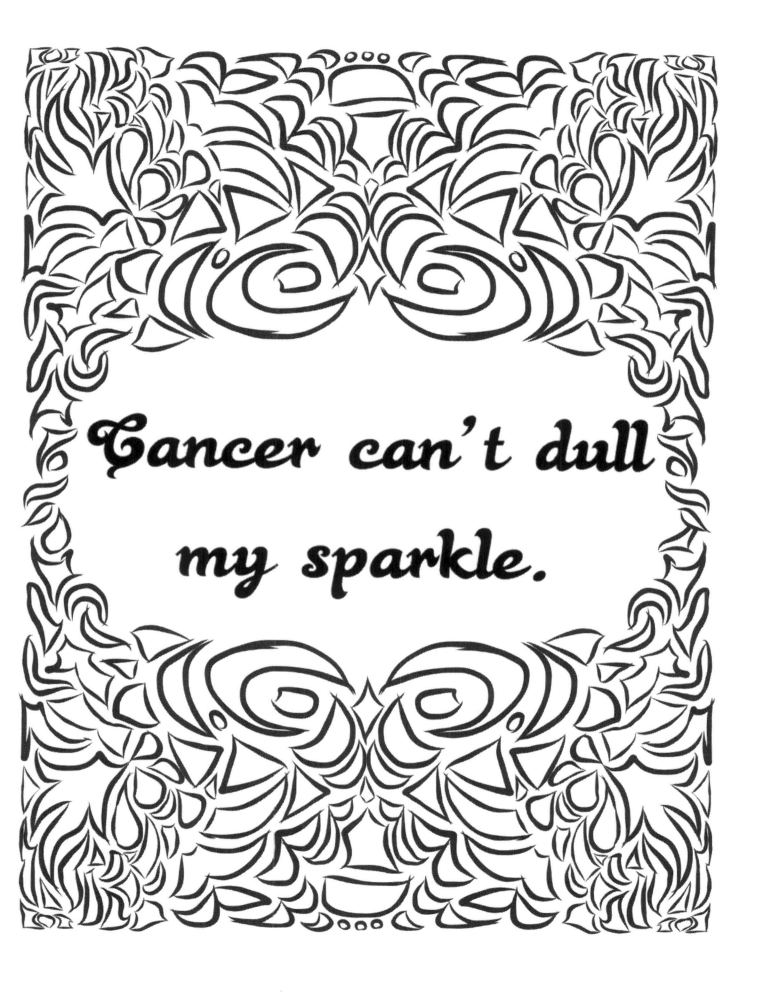

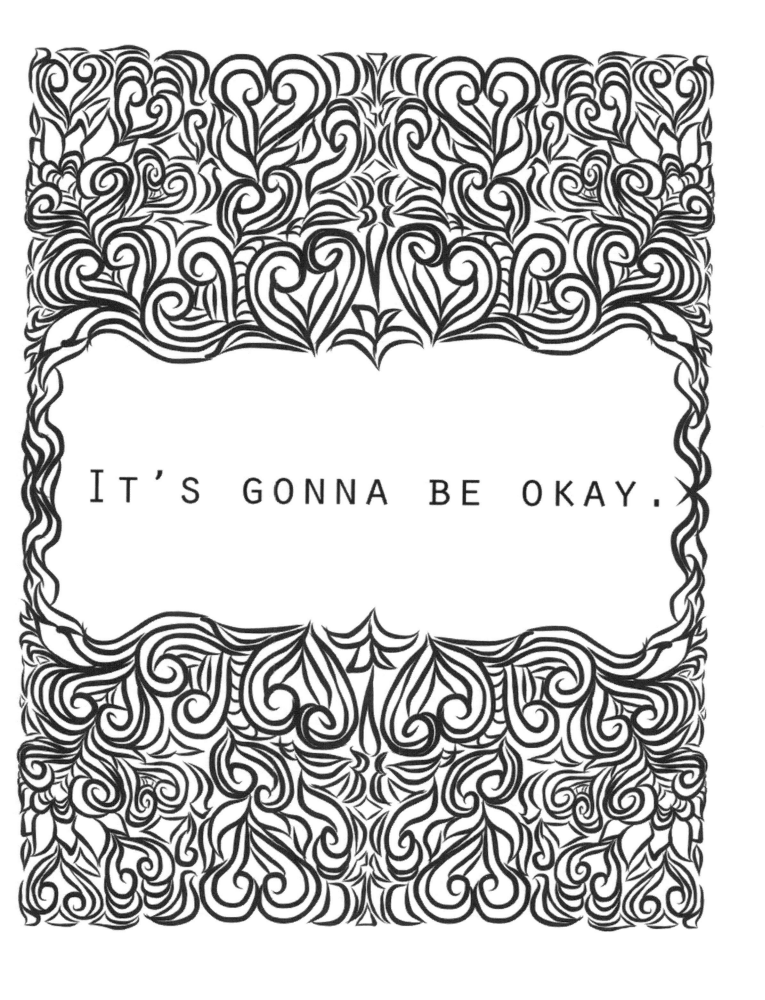

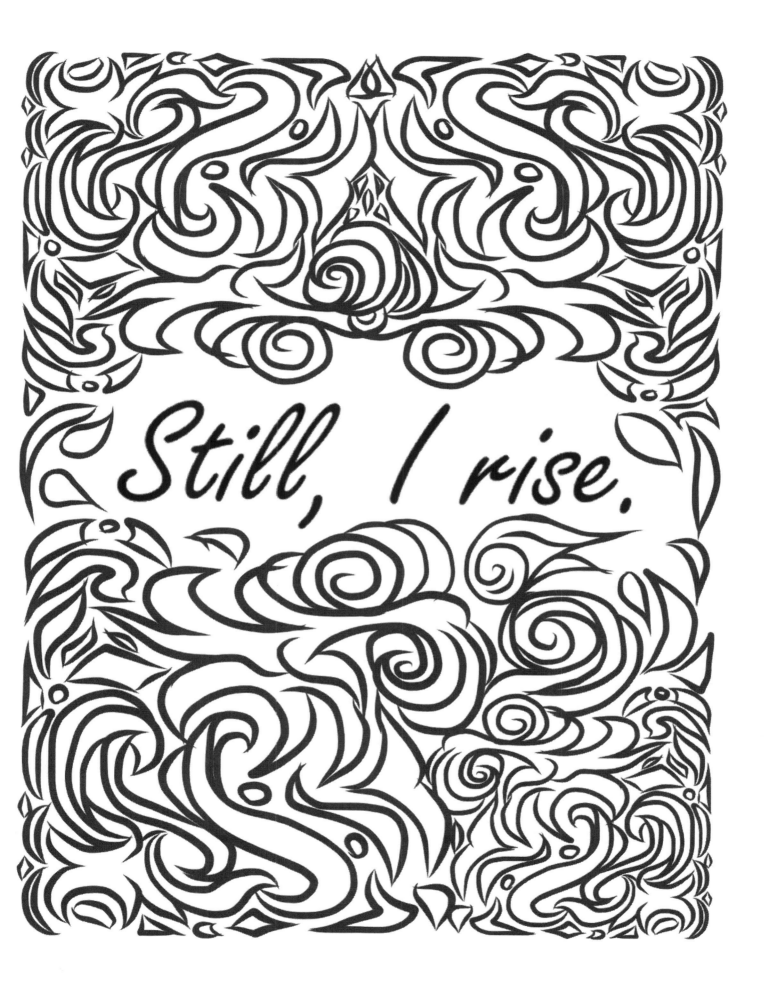

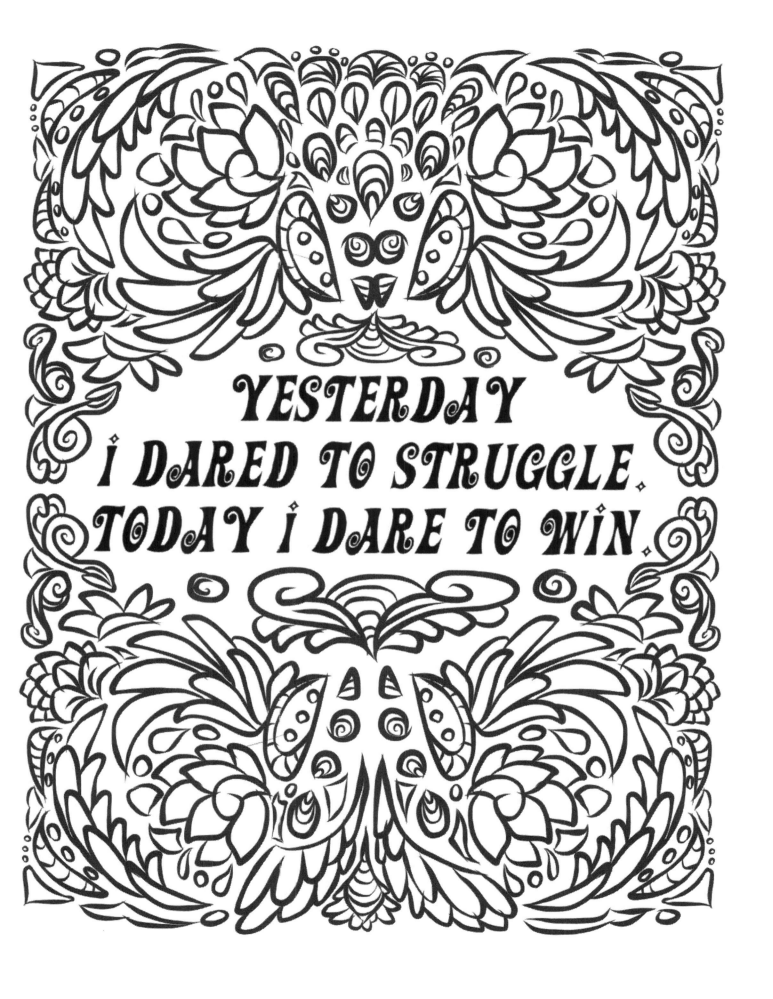

Made in the USA
Columbia, SC
21 February 2018